Unifying Human and Pet Nutraceutical Technology

Natures Benefit for Pets

Stephen Holt, M.D. and Dean R. Bader, DVM

With a Foreword by T.V. Taylor MD

Wellness Publishing Inc.
www.wellnesspublishing.com
Telephone Orders: 877-765-1099

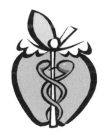

www.naturesbenefit.com

NATURES BENEIT FOR PETS

FOCUS ON SPECIFIC NUTRACEUTICALS

© Stephen Holt, M.D. and Dean R. Bader, DVM

Wellness Publishing Inc.
www.wellnesspublishing.com
75 Plymouth Street
Fairfield, NJ 07004
Tel. 877-765-1099

* SPECIAL NOTE: USE SUGGESTIONS IN THIS BOOK ONLY
WITH THE GUIDANCE OF A VETERINARIAN

ISBN 0-9714224-0-0

CONTENTS

Foreword

Human and veterinary medicine are closely linked. Drs. Holt and Bader pave the way to unifying human and pet nutritional sciences. This book is novel, and new in bridging the gap between natural medicine in humans and animals. It describes the thoughtful application of "human natural medicine" with nutraceuticals for pets. The word "nutraceutical" implies that nutrients (or natural products) have potential treatment properties. Accepting that advances in conventional medicine with drugs and surgery have contributed greatly to the treatment of disease in our pets, a new move exists to examine alternative, medical approaches. In the absence of a life threatening illness or medical emergency, many people have sought a natural medical option, before resorting to drugs or surgery. Humankind now sees the value of this approach for their cherished pets.

Not so long ago, there was "one" type of doctor. This doctor treated all creatures. The disciplines of human and veterinary medicine became well established in the 20th century, with the clear recognition of the special needs of various animal species. Not only did human and veterinary medicine split, but also specialized branches of medicine developed within these disciplines. Currently, there is a move back to the idea that there is "one type of medicine", but this type of medicine must be all embracing (eclectic).

The advent of a "blended" form of human and animal medicine was reported in the December issue (2000) of the Journal of the American Veterinary Medical Association. The lead, news article in this journal reported on a pivotal veterinary medical symposium entitled "The Bridge Between Veterinary Medicine and Human Health" (held in October 2000). This symposium was designed to bring together education and research from veterinary and human medicine. Clearly, there is great portability between animal and human health issues.

Whilst the vet is the obvious choice for overseeing pet health, a lot can be learned by transfer of knowledge from human medicine to veterinary medicine and vice versa. Given modern concepts of "unity of body function", it seems logical that we should now seek "unity" of medical knowledge. Dr. Holt is a physician with treatment experience limited to human medicine, where safety and efficacy issues are very challenging. Dr. Dean Bader is a holistic veterinarian who practices with a pluralistic approach involving conventional veterinary science. The authors are appropriately cautious to advise against "self-medication" by pet owners. They emphasize consistently that pet owners seek the advice of a licensed veterinarian. Our former quest for the "super specialist" in medicine has been replaced by our recognition of the importance of "holistic" care. These issues border on both conventional and alternative medical treatments - a circumstance that Dr. Holt describes as "medical pluralism" (or pluralistic medicine).

This book has been focused on "nutraceuticals" and it does not claim to be a complete account of animal health. However, it addresses many of the commonest, simple disorders that affect dogs, cats and horses. It does not contain advice to manage serious disease, which Drs. Holt and Bader demand be treated only by a veterinarian. What makes this book so refreshing and new is their pioneering attempt to bring advances in human natural medical therapies to our beloved pets, with the expert advice of a skilled, experienced veterinarian.

Dr. Stephen Holt is a physician, researcher and author par excellence. With eloquence, he describes the development of "nutraceuticals" (food or dietary supplements) for the care or adjunctive benefit of pets. Drawing upon their encyclopedic knowledge of medicine (animal and human), Drs. Holt and Bader describe the practical application of vital nutrients, herbs and botanicals in the management of wellness in pets. The benefits that exist in nature for animal and human well-being are obvious. They are intimately joined for application to humans and their companion animals.

Thomas V. Taylor, M.D.
Professor, Baylor College of Medicine
Professor, University of Texas
February 2001

Conventional and Natural Medicine Merges

There has been a revolution in healthcare over the past decade. High technology has merged with human and veterinary medicine. New drug development and refined surgical approaches have made great advances in disease treatment, but this "high tech" approach has failed predictably in several areas of wellness promotion. These days, humankind is seeking simpler, gentle and more natural approaches to disease prevention and treatment. We are moving into an era of medicine, which has become "pluralistic" in its approach. Remedies of natural origin such as nutrients, herbs and botanicals (nutraceuticals) have demonstrated safe and effective promises for wellness maintenance in all branches of medicine. Currently, there is a shifting treatment paradigm away from drug therapies for certain disorders in pets, especially given the frequent occurrence of serious or occasionally fatal side effects of pharmaceuticals.

There is growing self-reliance among healthcare consumers to seek natural approaches to health and well-being. Coincidental with this move is a greater tendency for people to self diagnose and self medicate. The notion of "medication" has been subjected to an expanded definition that now includes "remedies of natural origin". However, food supplements are not to be confused with drugs. Scientists now discuss "medicalized" foods, nutritional supplements and other natural substances along with drug treatments. In some circumstances, these natural remedies have replaced conventional (allopathic) treatments and in many cases they are used as adjunctive (additive) treatments with great benefits. This latter situation has led do the concept of complementary medicine in veterinary and human medical practice. "Complementary" is a term that is sometimes used synonymously with "alternative", "integrated" or "pluralistic", when describing "eclectic" forms of medicine.

While much media attention has focused on the emergence of "natural medicine" in humans, a natural healthcare revolution is occurring in veterinary medical practice. The recognition of "optimal" nutrition for "optimal" health in pets has led to massive interest in new diets for animals. Many pet foods are designed to have special health purposes. They are types of "functional food". These new diets are based on the principals of modern science and nutrition. Few healthcare givers deny the power of food as medicine, but not all apply this power.

Holistic care and eclectic treatments are used increasingly in veterinary practice. Our pets have instinctive drives to maintain their wellness by natural means. Examples of this circumstance abound in the animal kingdom. This book highlights the shifting treatment and healthcare paradigms in veterinary medicine. It examines natural approaches for the management of common health problems that face pet owners in the care and maintenance of wellness in their beloved companions. This book brings knowledge from human, nutraceutical advances that are readily applied with benefit to pets. It will surprise some readers to learn that several nutraceutical technologies have been developed by veterinary scientists, but these advances have enjoyed their greatest application in human medicine, rather than veterinary medicine.

Stephen Holt, M.D.
and
Dean R. Bader, DVM

Natural Ways to Bone and Joint Health

It seems like many pet owners have accepted the concept of the "old lame dog" (cat or horse). This is negative thinking, which should be extinguished. These days, "creaky joints" from arthritis or hip dysplasia need not be perceived as an inevitability. Scientific advances in nutritional and botanical support for bone and joint health have made a real difference to the mobility and well-being of our loved companions. There are many advances in remedies of natural origin for bone and joint health in humans that are now being applied to dogs, cats and horses.

Popular remedies of natural origin for joint disorders

Well-controlled clinical observations demonstrate clearly that remedies of natural origin can effectively improve the symptoms of arthritis or stress injuries to joints. More than a "quick fix" for symptom relief, several of these natural agents may go to the root of the problems in arthritis. Many of these issues are covered in the book *The Power of Cartilage* (Kensington NY, 1998), authors, S. Holt and J. Barilla.

So important and neglected are these agents that they are now prominently summarized in Table 1.

Glucosamine: or glycoaminoglycans (GAG) have been shown in prospective clinical studies to improve symptoms and signs of arthritis and assist in regeneration of joint cartilage.

Chondroitin: similar actions to glucosamine, with a common anti-inflammatory effect, but variably absorbed from the gut.

Shark cartilage (researched as Cartilade, Cartivet and Cartequine): a holistic mixture of glucosamine-like components (glycoaminoglycans), chondroitin, type II collagen, calcium, phosphorous (2:1 ratio), and antiangiogenic proteins.

Hydrolyzed collagen: type II collagen of bovine, shark, or chicken origin is effective in arthritis (especially inflammatory arthritis or rheumatoid disease) by mechanisms of immune tolerance.

Bromelain: enzymes that take care of soft tissue injury and inflammation.

Boswellia serrata: a natural anti-inflammatory with actions somewhat similar to NSAIDs, without any gastrointestinal side effects.

Methylsulphonylmethane (MSM): a sulphur containing natural anti-inflammatory with credible evidence of improvements in pain and inflammation in joints.

Green-lipped mussel: contains GAG and other natural anti-inflammatory substances.

Others: cetyl myristate, ginger, sea cucumber, with evidence of benefit in arthritis and joint problems.

Table 1
Arthritis and other bone and joint disorders. These agents are reviewed in detail later.

The remedies of natural origin listed in Table 1 are often used as safe and quite effective alternatives to drugs in holistic vet practice. One drawback, however, is that these natural agents, with the exception of Boswellia and perhaps MSM, take time to be effective (between 2 and 12 weeks). The delay in onset of several natural remedies in an important concept to understand in natural medicine. Failure to recognize the delay sometimes results in premature abandonment of nutraceutical approaches.

Drugs versus Natural Therapies

The drug treatment of arthritis with non-steroidal anti-inflammatory drugs (NSAID) and corticosteroids possesses many disadvantages and limitations. In conventional veterinary practice, the use of anti-inflammatory, pain-killing medication produces short-lived effects; and it is associated with serious side effects in pets. Extensive medical research over the past 30 years has shown that NSAID cause life threatening bleeding from the gastrointestinal tract, interference with kidney function and they often cause liver damage. What happens with NSAID usage in humans happens also in our pets. Dr. Holt and his colleagues reported in 1989 that 62% of all patients admitted to three different hospitals with bleeding from the upper digestive tract were taking NSAID (e.g. ibuprofen, naproxen, suldinac, indomethacin etc.). Furthermore, NSAID cause bleeding from the lower digestive tract and they may cause a "leaky gut". A leaky gut (enhanced permeability of the intestines) contributes to many illnesses and it can increase the occurrence of food allergies.

Of particular importance is the recognition that many of these "anti-arthritic" medications tend to cause serious problems most often in the elderly. The elderly comprise the target population who most frequently use these drugs. Older humans and animals tend to have "thin bones and creaky joints" (osteoporosis and osteoarthritis, OA). Just as elderly humans receive NSAID, it is elderly pets who also commonly receive these drugs. Elderly pets and humans are very vulnerable to the side effects of NSAID. We reinforce the impressive evidence of the dangers of NSAID therapy in humans, because the same situations occur in dogs, cats and horses; but the amount of follow-up information on NSAID usage that has been collected in animals is less than that described in humans.

Added to these problems with NSAID is the experimental evidence that certain NSAID may actually damage the cartilage in the joints of dogs. This is of particular concern because damage to cartilage is the basic mechanism of common types of arthritis in animals and humans (osteoarthritis, OA). The dangers of the chronic use of steroids (cortisone, corticosteroids) in animals require no discussion. Corticosteroids have "no role" in the treatment of osteoarthritis, because of their questionable effectiveness and serious side effects. Side effects of steroids for the treatment of osteoarthritis are so severe that they outweigh any long-term benefit from their use. In addition, the popular use of phenylbutazone ("Bute") in horses is sometimes associated with severe and life threatening complications.

TV commercials that promoted the use of certain NSAID in dogs were dropped by pharmaceutical companies, when they were told by Government agencies to warn about "death" as a side effect of certain NSAID drugs. So serious and pernicious are the side effects of these anti-arthritic drugs that many people have sought natural alternatives for bone and joint health (Table 1). Recent research indicates that a number of specific nutrients and natural agents (herbal and botanicals) can be used effectively to help prevent and manage arthritis or bone and joint problems in pets in a safe, simple and cost-effective manner (Table 1).

Types of arthritis and their diagnosis

The commonest types of "arthritis" encountered in dogs include hip dysplasia; elbow dysplasia, osteoarthritis and bone or soft tissue and joint disruption from "stress injury". Similar conditions occur in cats and horses. Acute stress injury is very common in competitive animals (e.g. greyhounds, racehorses, polo-horses, jumpers etc.). Sometimes the manifestation of arthritis is obvious in our pets. They present with a slow gait, a limp, reduced mobility or lameness. Most often the signs of arthritis are subtler, such as reduced spontaneous activity and slowness in the initiation of exercise. Bone and joint problems in competitive animals are the commonest reason for them to slow down in events. Sometimes our loved companions just "suffer in silence". Anyone who experiences the pain of arthritis or acute skeletal injury can understand the dreadful concept of "suffering in silence".

Arthritis in its most common form is a disease of cartilage in joints. Cartilage is a spongy substance that permits joints to move without much friction. Many natural therapies protect cartilage from damage or they can help repair damaged cartilage. The repair, renewal and regeneration of cartilage are a big issue in natural medicine. When arthritis becomes advanced, soft tissue problems, such as thickening of the lining of joints, reduced range of movement of the joint and foreign body accumulation within the joints may all be present.

In established arthritis new blood vessels grow into joints. This process is called angiogenesis (angio=blood vessel, genesis=growth). Substances that interfere with this unwanted blood vessel growth (angiogenesis) are called antiangiogenic compounds (see discussions of shark cartilage).

Soft tissue problems are often overlooked in arthritic animals and nutraceuticals should ideally contain antioxidants e.g. vitamin C, an antioxidant, or enzymes i.e. bromelain that assist in the resolution of soft tissue problems. Arthritic changes can be easily felt in joints. If a hand is gently placed on an arthritic joint or dysplastic joint, a "crackling sensation" in the joint may be apparent. This is a common clinical sign called "crepitus". Sometimes with passive movement of an arthritic joint, the "cracking" can be loud enough to be heard.

There is a never-ending debate in veterinary medicine about whether hereditary or other factors such as "wear and tear" cause common arthritis in dogs and cats (see discussions about hip dysplasia). On occasion dogs suffer from inflammatory types of joint disease where joints are "hot" and painful. This disorder is sometimes related to acute injury or disordered immunity or occasionally infection. Infected joints are an acute emergency, requiring antibiotic therapy, but inflammatory arthritis, similar to the human disease of rheumatoid arthritis, can occur infrequently in cats, dogs or horses.

Many veterinarians have stressed the importance of the accurate diagnosis of arthritis. This subject has been covered in detail by Dr. Shawn Messonier DVM in his excellent book entitled "The Arthritis Solution". Occasionally other diseases, such as cancer, cause lameness and there are many different types of arthritis, which may require specific treatments. However, by far the commonest type of arthritis is osteoarthritis (OA) and this review focuses upon this problem. In all cases of doubt pet owners must seek the advice of their veterinarian. A proper diagnosis is an absolute prerequisite for effective treatment.

The importance of nutrition

The optimal diet for bone and joint health includes adequate calcium, phosphorus, protein and essential fatty acids. Several practitioners of alternative or holistic veterinary medicine have emphasized the role of "cooked food" in the causation of arthritis. Feeding animals nutritious, "raw" food, which is enriched with digestive enzymes, may benefit some animals, but the principal issue to be addressed is often the presence of optimal digestive health. Optimal digestive health can be assisted by the administration of enzymes and probiotics (friendly bacteria) and several supplements are available to add to food in a convenient manner (see section 6 on Digestive Health).

The best nutraceutical approach to digestive health is the comprehensive use of probiotics (friendly bacteria) with prebiotics (factors that cause friendly bacteria to grow), enzymes (to assist digestion) and specific herbals that can assist in detoxification (e.g. Milk Thistle). Creaky joints go hand in hand with thin bones and added sources of dietary calcium are often important for optimal bone and joint health. Calcium is found in plentiful amounts in Cartivet Plus and Cartequine Plus, but it is absent in many other nutraceuticals for joints (e.g. Cosequin, Glycoflex, Cosamin etc.).

Dietary supplements (Nutraceuticals)

Pet owners have been impressed by the use of glucosamine with or without chondroitin and trace minerals for joint disorders, but many new and exciting natural agents for bone and joint health have appeared with good evidence for their benefit (Table 1). Few pet owners realize that the research on glucosamine and chondroitin came originally from observations of the benefits of feeding cartilage to dogs, cats and horses (Table 2). In fact, cartilage supplements form the most holistic of all supplements for bone and joint health, because of their content of glycoaminoglycans (glucosamine-like compounds), chondroitin, calcium, phosphorus, type II collagen, trace minerals and antiangiogenic protein (Table 2).

Component	Therapeutic Potential
Calcium and Phosphorus in a 2:1 ratio	Ideal, balanced, bioavailable mineral supplement for bones (prevents osteoporosis).
Collagen, Type II	A nutrient with potential for the development of the immune tolerance phenomenon (e.g. rheumatoid and connective tissue disease).
Antiangiogenic Protein	Varying molecular weight antiangiogenic proteins have been repeatedly demonstrated in shark cartilage. The molecular weight of some of these proteins is such that they may cross the intestinal mucosal barrier. Potential action in many angiogenesis-dependent diseases, e.g. cancer, arthritis, skin disease, proliferative retinopathy, Kaposis sarcoma.
Glucosamine-like compounds Chondroitin sulfate Heparan sulfate, Dermatan sulfate, Keratan sulfate, etc.	Regarded as potential therapy for arthritis.

Table 2
Constituents of shark cartilage that may confer a health benefit in several disease states. Potential mechanisms of actions and applications are summarized.

Supplements that contain glucosamine and chondroitin with trace elements (e.g. Cosequine, Cosamin etc.) have been superseded by new, more complex combinations of natural agents that have the promise of being much more effective than glucosamine and chondroitin plus minerals alone e.g. Cartivet-Plus, Cartequine Plus and others (Table 3). Exciting natural substances such as methylsulphonylmethane (MSM), Boswellia serrata and Green-lipped mussel can be used in combination with glucosamine, cartilage supplements and trace elements to provide the ultimate holistic combination of natural products for the prevention and treatment of bone and joint problems in dogs (Table 3). This is the complete and holistic formulation for bone and joint health for dogs, cats and horses (Table 3).

	Dose Range	
Glucosamine 2KCL Sulphate	1 g	2 g
Hydrolyzed Collagen	0.5 g	1 g
Methylsulfonylmethane (MSM)	0.2 g	0.4 g
Boswellia serrata	0.1 g	0.2 g
Bromelain (enzymes)	37.8 mg	75.6 mg
Vitamin C	0.5 g	1 g
Shark Cartilage (100% pure Cartilade)	1.05 g	2.1 g
Brewers Yeast	0.5 g	1 g
New Zealand Green Lipped Mussel	0.1 g	0.2 g

Table 3
Ingredient and amounts in holistic bone and joint formulae
supplied by permission of Nature's Benefit, Inc.

Eclectic approaches to bone and joint health

Topical therapy (surface application) with essential oils (aromatherapy), homeopathic agents and capsicum derivatives (peppers) are valuable in the acute relief of joint problems. These natural approaches are additive therapies for use with dietary (food) supplements. Chiropractic and "touch therapies" are very valuable approaches for arthritic problems or stress injuries, as are acupuncture, acupressure and massage performed by skilled individuals.

Certain "physical" treatments are very useful in acute and chronic care of musculoskeletal problems. Recent research with magnetic therapy, preferably using moving electromagnetic fields, and targeted hydrotherapy have shown great promise in improving mobility in elderly animals. Finally, the environment in which your pet lives is very important. Warm, dry, comforting beds with lots of attention and love are effective healing influences. The arthritic dog should not be stressed by separation anxiety and unnecessary excitement or "giddiness" (see sections 5, Behavioral Problems). Natural remedies that allay anxiety and calm your pet in times of stress have to be considered. Most important, we must not let our pets "suffer in silence".

Introducing cartilage supplements

Pets, like people, have ailments and injuries that can be helped with the use of cartilage supplements. There are numerous studies in dogs, cats, and horses that have demonstrated the benefits of cartilage on various conditions that affect animals and humans (see the book, The Power of Cartilage, Kensington Publishing, NY, 1998). Supplements of cartilage from cows, chickens and sharks have well described benefits in animals with bone and joint problems. Dr. Shawn Messonier DVM has discussed the benefit of cartilage supplements in his book "The Arthritis Solution for Dogs" (Prima Publishing, CA, 2000).

The rationale for the use of shark cartilage in several disease states has been largely based on the knowledge that it is an ideal holistic mixture of glycoaminoglycans (glucosamine-like compounds), chondroitin, type II collagen, calcium, phosphorus, trace elements and antiangiogenic proteins (Table 2). Cartilage administered to animals and humans in varying formats and dosages may exert an anti-angiogenic effect. Antiangiogenesis is interference with unwanted blood vessel growth (anti=against, angio=blood vessel, genesis-growth). Angiogenesis (the growth of new blood vessels) is an underlying mechanism associated with a variety of diseases, including cancer, arthritis, proliferative retinopathy, neovascular glaucoma, and skin diseases, such as psoriasis (see section 9, Liposome Angio-Inhibitor).

In the September-October 1994 issue of Natural Pet, Dr. Ben Dow, a Vermont veterinarian, told readers how a beautiful collie was saved from the "jaws of death". The animal was crippled with arthritis and could hardly walk. Dr. Dow had tried conventional drugs and therapies to no avail. Having heard about shark cartilage and its effects on arthritis for humans, he decided to give it a try. After about two weeks, the owners called. Dr. Dow expected they would again ask to have the dog put down. But the report would not ask to have the dog put down. But the report was that the collie was running up and down the stairs, playing with the cat and even jumping into the owners' pickup truck! " I began to use shark cartilage (Cartivet) for dogs with arthritis and also dogs and cats with tumors. I am happy to report that the results have been very encouraging", said Dr. Dow.

Some scientists believe that cartilage has other beneficial effects in a variety of disease states. These effects are attributed to substances in cartilage that have direct effects on immune function. Elegant scientific work exists in animal experiments that show cartilage therapy may assist in the induction of immune tolerance in arthritis (see type II collagen), especially in forms of arthritis that have a basis in disordered immune function. Certain fractions of cartilage, such as Glucosamine-like compounds (glycosaminoglycans, GAG), have been shown to have beneficial effects in arthritis with benefits similar to non-steroidal anti-inflammatory drugs (NSAID). However, natural anti-inflammatory substances like glucosamine and glycoaminoglycans in cartilage often take between 2 and 12 weeks to be maximally beneficial. Shark cartilage may contain up to 12% of chondroitin sulfate, which has also been proposed as an effective remedy for arthritis. Whilst, these results are promising, less research work has been done with natural agents compared with drug treatments.

Cartilage for bone and joint health

Animal studies indicate that shark cartilage shows promise in the treatment of arthritis and other inflammatory joint disorders. These clinical studies in animals have shown quite promising results with the use of cartilage for the treatment of arthritis of diverse form. Very important data comes from a presentation made by Dr. J. Rauis at the British Small Animal Veterinary Association Congress (1991). Dr. Rauis reported on the beneficial effects of shark cartilage in treating dogs with secondary arthritis. Dr. Rauis treated ten dogs with lameness due to the following disorders alone or in combination: joint fracture (2), hip dysplasia(4), joint dislocation (2), spondylopathy (2), and rupture of the cruciate ligament (2). The presence of osteoarthritis was confirmed by X-ray and other tests in all animals. Each dog received 1 capsule of Cartilage (740 milligrams) per 5 kilograms of body weight per day for 3 weeks.

Evaluations of the dogs were made at days 0, 8, 15, 21, and 30 of the study, and clinical scores of disability were made regularly. Each of several clinical disabilities or measures of mobility in the dogs was charted with special reference to lameness. These parameters included: local swelling, atrophy (shrinkage) of regional muscles, joint crepitation and/or pain, lameness before action, lameness after action, and difficulty in negotiating an obstacle. Lameness was clearly defined as difficulty in walking or running after several hours of immobility (lameness before action), lameness involving the climbing of stairs and/or the capacity to get over an obstacle that had not been previously overcome by the animal.

There were several striking beneficial outcomes in this study by Dr. Rauis. Of note, were no significant side effects and the shark cartilage was considered very easy to administer to the dogs. It mixed readily with dog meals, and nine out of then animals were reported to "like" it very much. In all cases, the owners indicated that their dogs were much more active and even "happy". The impression of happiness was ascribed to pain relief in the dogs. The main beneficial effect seemed to be reduction in local swelling and inflammation in the dogs' joints. The overall effect on functional parameters in the dogs was described as "impressive" by Dr. Rauis.

The owners of the dogs had comments to make about the treatment. Ada, a 7-year old Labrador female, had very pronounced hip dysplasia and had received surgery for a torn knee ligament. She moved slowly and needed help to climb stairs. Her knee creaked when she walked. After treatment, her owner said that Ada was "*much more alive, more happy.*"

Tob, a 14-year old crossbreed male, was obese, had hip joint dislocation, could not jump or climb stairs, and was in pain with movement. After treatment, his owner said the dog was "*much more mobile, seemed to be very happy, and [he] climbs stairs alone and jumps.*" Zorro, a 16-year old male poodle, had hip dysplasia with chronic dislocation of one joint. He walked with difficulty and movement was very painful. After treatment his owner reported that there was "*very spectacular*" improvement already by the second day of treatment. "*Zorro is much better. He walks normally, climbs stairs, and runs some distance.*" Moritz, a Labrador male, had been off shark cartilage for 4 weeks. His owner noted that the improvement in osteoarthritis has lasted for 2 weeks and then decreased, but not completely. After 3 weeks of the second course of cartilage supplements, the improvement was better than after three weeks of the first treatment.

No.	Breed	Sex	Age, Years	Condition	Results at 30 Days
1	Miniature Schnauzer	ME	12	Arthritis	Poor compliance
2	Cross terrier	FN	15	Arthritis	Poor compliance
3	Petit basset griffon Vendeen	FN	13	Arthritis	Improved
4	Border collie	FN	9	Arthritis, right hindleg	Good
5	Old English sheepdog	ME	12	Arthritis and neoplasia	Euthanized
6	Shetland sheepdog	ME	11.25	Arthritis in elbows	Improved
7	Old English sheepdog	FE	15	Arthritis and mammary neoplasia	Good
8	Cavalier King Charles spaniel	FE	7.8	Spondylosis	Good
9	German shepherd	FN	9.9	Hip dysplasia and arthritis	Poor
10	Basset hound	ME	9.5	Generalized arthritis	Poor compliance
11	Lhasa apso	ME	8.2	Arthritis, hips	Euthanized
12	Old English sheepdog	ME	11.3	Arthritis and neoplasia	Improved

Table 4

Clinical features and overall outcome of twelve dogs with degenerative joint disease that were treated with CartiVet™ (100% pure shark cartilage) by Dr. Trevor Turner DVM (1996), former President of the British Small Animal Veterinary Association.

Recent studies of the use of 100% pure shark cartilage product by Dr. Trevor Turner DVM in England, confirm earlier observations (Table 4). Dr. Turner (1996) reported a series of 12 dogs with osteoarthritis and solid tumors (3 of 12 cases) in the British journal of Veterinary Practice News. All animals in this series were suffering from osteoarthritis in one or more limbs and two of the dogs had dysplasia (Table 4). Each of the animals had received treatment with conventional therapy, including non-steroidal anti-inflammatory drugs, analgesics, or corticosteroids, with limited benefits. This group of animals was regarded as experiencing circumstances of failure of conventional, veterinary therapies.

The dogs received 1 gram per 7 kilograms of body weight of shark cartilage product, and if improvement was observed in the trial, conventional medication was reduced. Only 9 of the 12 animals were able to be evaluated because of noncompliance in three cases. Of these 9 animals, 3 (33%) showed good improvement and 3 (33%) showed definite signs of some improvement after 30days of treatment with shark cartilage product. Only one dog failed to respond and two dogs were euthanized. Dr. Turner commented on the owners' enthusiasm to continue the product where improvement had occurred and stressed the absence of side effects with the use of the shark cartilage product. Based on these results, Dr. Turner concluded that shark cartilage product has a place among alternative medicines in the treatment of osteoarthritis (degenerative joint disease) in dogs and cats. More studies are justified to assess the potential benefits of shark cartilage for cancer.

Cartilage supplements in horses

The current trend in medicine, both for animals and humans, is a general movement away from synthetic drugs toward more natural products. A holistic approach to preventing and treating disease is being accepted and incorporated into modern health care. A nutraceutical that seems to please many pet owners and vets (traditional or holistic) is shark cartilage. Well-prepared shark cartilage is not chemically altered or contaminated and its use has a sound scientific basis. Practitioners of many disciplines of human health care, like many veterinarians, believe shark cartilage to be extremely useful, by virtue of its nutrient profile.

Powdered shark cartilage seems to offer hope and promise in reducing the symptoms associated with chronic inflammation of bone, joints, connective tissues, and other conditions. It has been demonstrated to have a direct application for use in injuries and other exercised-related discomforts suffered by horses as well in relievening stiffness and pain among elderly horses.

There have been several, clinical studies of the effects of shark cartilage (Cartequine® and CartiVet®) on horses and small animals, respectively. A British, clinical trial studied the benefits of Cartequine® in the reduction of pain and enhancement of mobility in horses at the Home for Rest Horses (Speen Farm, Bucks, England). This trial involved thirty horses with a variety of mobility problems, including non-specific lameness and degenerative joint disease. These horses were selected for study from one hundred elderly, retired, injured, or abandoned horses at the Home of Rest. The beneficial results of this trial in improving mobility were very promising in these elderly horses with joint problems.

Many horses have been entered in the Olympics and other major competitive events while taking shark cartilage (Cartequine). Geoff Billington, Olympic competitor and noted British jockey and trainer, feeds his horses shark cartilage (Cartequine) regularly for several weeks before competitive events He endorses the use of shark cartilage to treat horses with skeletal problems. He used Cartequine® as a natural mobility supplement for his horse Otto which entered and was placed in the Olympics held in Atlanta in 1996. In addition, Billington reported that his horse Manouso, who won the puissance event at the Horse of the Year Show in Wembley, England in 1996, did very well on Cartequine®, as a natural alternative to phenylbutazone ("Bute"). Phenylbutazone ("Bute") has onerous side effects.

Some jockeys have reported that the anti-inflammatory effects of shark cartilage are as good as those experienced with anti-inflammatory drugs. The British Federation Equestrian International has said that Cartequine® may be used in competition, while butazolidin ("Bute") has been banned. The Jockey Club in the UK has indicated that Cartequine® contains no substances that are "prohibited," so animals can continue, "to run" when using the supplement Cartequine®. Cartequine was described as helping competitive horses "stay in the race".

Gregory L. Ferraro, D.V.M., an equine (horse) practitioner of orthopedic medicine and surgery, with more than 25 years at Southern California racetracks, believes that shark cartilage (Cartequine) may benefit horses because of its anti-inflammatory properties. Shark cartilage appears to have the potential of providing horse owners with a powerful, natural anti-inflammatory agent that avoids the problems that are so often associated with the use of conventional anti-inflammatory drugs. Dr. Ferraro, who is an Associate Professor of Equine Surgery at the University of California at Davis School of Veterinary Medicine, performed a landmark study of Cartequine (100% pure shark cartilage) in competitive racehorses.

To determine whether shark cartilage would benefit horses, Dr. Ferraro conducted a clinical study of seven competitive thoroughbreds. The study group consisted of three females and four males, age range 3-6 years. (See Table 5) This study was undertaken to determine the tolerability and effectiveness of 100% shark cartilage (Cartequine®) in the treatment of common joint problems in the athletic horse. The horses were selected from three different training stables in California and all were in active, daily training and periodic competition. Although the horses were in good general health and were deemed "racing sound," each suffered from mild to moderate degrees of osteoarthritis or degenerative joint change in two or more joints (Table 5).

Each horse underwent an examination prior to entry into the study and on a weekly basis thereafter for eight weeks. The animals received 10 grams daily of 100% pure shark cartilage for 10 days, followed by 5 grams daily for an additional 50 days. During the study, the horses remained on a daily training regimen and each animal was monitored daily for general well-being, appetite, and any adverse effects of the study medication (Table 5). The clinical status for each horse is summarized in Table 5.

DR. GREGORY FERRARO'S LANDMARK STUDY ON CARTEQUINE IN COMPETITIVE HORSES SHOWED GREAT BENEFIT. HORSES COULD "STAY IN THE RACE."

Clinical Status Prior to Study

4 yr. Old stallion in continuous training for 12 months prior to study.

A "stakes-class" racehorse who suffered from OA in both front fetlocks with moderate to severe bouts of capsulitis.

4 yr. Old gelding in continuous training for seven months, had undergone carpal surgery to remove a chrondial fracture one year prior to study. The animal had moderate amount of joint distention and osteoarthritis in capri.

4 yr. old filly in training 10 months prior to the study, raced in "allowance" type race, a slight to moderate amount of joint inflammation as a result of of "tying up".

4 yr. old filly in continuous training of both fetlocks due to chronic osteoarthri tis in both joints, a "stakes" class individual.

4 yr. old stallion in continuous training for 9 mo. Prior to clinical investigation, had history of a surgical repair of a non-displaced lateral condylar fracture of the distal metacarpus 17 months prior to study, moderate amount of joint disten tion and capsulitis as result of chronic osteoarthritis in both front fetlocks, an "allowance" level competitor.

Clinical Progress and End Point Comments

Slight improvement in clinical appearance of Fetlock joints and training performance by third week of study, continued to steadily improve over second month of investigation and had fewer non-training days during this Period.
Periodic treatments with phenylbutazone, which were necessary before the shark cartilage therapy began, were discontinued.

No improvement during first month of study, the inflammation and distention in fetlock joints worsened during the first 2-3 weeks of trial; by second month this animal began to show steady improvement. Shark cartilage Therapy had no effect, on post-trial exercise myositis ("tying up").

Remarkable improvement by second week of study, chronic carpal inflammation and joint distention disappeared and training soundness also improved. By the third osteoarthritis, also intermittent bouts week of study, removed from daily regimen Of oral Butazolidin, continued to improve clinically over course of investigation and it was unnecessary to dose with NSAID, in spite of more intensified training.

Only slight improvement in fetlock for 9 months prior to study. Capsulitis inflammation until the fourth week of investigation. At that time began to show market decrease in joint effusion and Capsulitis, improved steadily over four weeks.

Improvement began to become apparent by the third week of the program, exhibited a moderate reduction of joint distention and pain at the time and maintained that state throughout the rest of the study period.

5 yr. old gelding in continuous training for 10 mo. Prior to trial, had history of carpal surgery to remove osteochrondial fracture 18 mos. Prior. Joint showed no evidence of chronic inflammation, exhibited problems of osteoarthritis of both front fetlocks with capsulitis and joint effusion, "stakes" class competitor.

During the first 10 day period of 10g/day of Cartequine, this animal showed immediate improvement, improved state lessened when dosage was decreased to 5 g/day, but joint inflammation did again show improvement in the fourth week and continued to improve thereafter.

Table 5
Clinical status of individual horses treated with Cartequine™, a 100% pure, shark cartilage preparation.

The clinical outcome results of Dr. Ferraro were based on daily clinical examinations and subjective assessments of physical status. Overall, the results indicated a beneficial therapeutic effect for shark cartilage product. Of the 70% of horses who responded, in this study by Dr. Ferrarro, *many needed 17 to 21 days of treatment before they showed maximum improvement in symptoms*. During the second month of the trial, the group as a whole appeared less bothered by their orthopedic disease, trained better, and required less use of other anti-inflammatory therapies. Overall, shark cartilage supplementation produced an average of 59% improvement. Positive changes were noted in many of the horses, *including decreases in joint and tendon swelling and inflammation, improved general mobility, and performance, improvement in skin and coat condition, and increase in rate of hoof growth.* Dr. Ferrarro notes that these are significant levels of response for any medication administered to "athletes-in-training" who may have long-standing or significant, "soundness" problems.

According to Dr. Ferrarro, there were no adverse reactions, dietary upsets, or detrimental effects from Cartequine observed in any horse involved in the study. All of the horses ate the product freely, without negative effects on appetite. Shark cartilage thus appears to be an economically sound, natural alternative for the management of the results of general wear and tear on horses' joints. The results of this clinical study indicated that shark cartilage has become one of the standards of natural treatments for bone and joint problems encountered in the competitive horse.

The Ecology of Sharks

Sharks are a precious part of Nature. How does one reconcile the use of this resource even with the knowledge that shark cartilage and other derivatives of sharks have valuable application in veterinary and human medicine? The most important issue is to avoid shark material that has been obtained by irresponsible fishing practices and to utilize material that is already part of the food chain. Shark "steaks" are popular in many countries and the meat of a shark is a high quality, low cholesterol source of protein. In fact, shark is very popular in Western Europe with the affinity of the British for "fish and chips".

The shark cartilage material used by responsible, nutraceutical companies must come from practices that do not disturb the ecology. Unfortunately, not all shark is derived in this manner. If a supplier cannot reassure people about the responsible collection of the material, then the use of suspect shark products must be boycotted. These are strong words, but responsible suppliers will not use or recommend any shark material that is collected in an irresponsible manner, without due concern for the depletion of shark species.

Marine Medicinals

Often, in our quest for newer and higher technology, we lose sight of the importance of natural resources. Like the rain forest, the ocean is a treasure chest of nutrients and substances with medicinal potential. We have only scratched the surface when it comes to harvesting health from the sea. Considering the usefulness of cartilage, shark oil, and shark meat, and the knowledge we can derive from studying immunity and detoxification systems, the shark is a virtual warehouse of health-giving substances. The ocean and lakes are teeming with other potential sources of nutrients: cold water fish with their omega-3 fatty acid (EPA and DHA) content; algae such as chlorella and spirulina dense with protein, minerals, and vitamins; and a host of other microorganisms. The recent massive interest in the supply of balanced minerals from "Coral Calcium" is a contemporary example of the value of marine nutraceuticals.

A recent article in *Trends in Biotechnology* (Vol. 15, September 1997) reported on the latest discoveries in "marine biotechnology"

– the vast potential of the oceans to lead to new cures for human and animal disease. William Fenical of the Center for Marine Biotechnology and Biomedicine, Scripps Institution of Oceanography, University of California-San Diego, explains that the growing incidence of drug-resistant infectious disease is a major incentive for finding new medicinals. Academic institutions and pharmaceutical companies are collaborating to "harvest" the fruits of the world's oceans. Hundreds of bioactive substances have been discovered in sponges, marine bacteria and fungi, and other marine plants and animals. These new compounds have potential as anti-inflammatory and anticancer "drugs". As with the shark, unlocking the secrets of these other inhabitants of the ocean will contribute to enhanced health for humankind.

A Plea: Reiterated

Sharks are precious creatures that should be treated with respect. The increasing recognition of the medicinal benefits of shark material should prompt good fishing practices. Do not use shark material if you know that it has come from irresponsible sources. Shark conservation is an important issue for the next millennium. A depletion of the shark population will have negative effects on marine ecology. If sharks are lost to us, a wealth of potential health benefits is also lost. At one time, the forerunner products to Cartequine and CartiVet were awarded endorsements by the Cousteau Society and a special award by the Prime minister of Costa Rica. The reason for mentioning the type of shark cartilage used in studies is because the major variations in shark material quality, purity and biological activity.

Summing Up on Shark Cartilage

Much evidence exists to support the potential benefits of shark cartilage as a dietary supplement to promote bone joint health in small animals and horses. Cartilage extracts or analogues of extracts, such as glucosamine, chondroitin, and collagen hydrolysates, may be effective in arthritis; and they assist in the promotion of skeletal health. However, complete formats of cartilage are often preferred over fractions containing GAG and or chondroitin, because they represent a more holistic approach to therapy. Whole cartilage is more cost-effective than isolated fractions alone. Users of cartilage preparations are advised to examine the research background upon which a particular brand of cartilage is sold. One clear and obvious benefit of shark cartilage is its content of calcium and phosphorus in an ideal ratio of 2:1, together with a wide range of vital trace minerals. The presence of variability among cartilage means that safety and effectiveness may not be portable between brands. Overall, shark cartilage therapy for animals (as well as for humans) appears to be very versatile in its actions on maintaining bone and joint health. It forms the basis upon which one can build leading-edge nutraceutical interventions for skeletal health in animals.

The development of holistic bone and joint formulae

Whilst it is clear that more than a decade of shark cartilage (and bovine and chicken cartilage) research has shown benefits of these nutraceuticals for bone and joint health, other natural bone and joint health products have been developed that have versatile, positive benefits when added to shark cartilage. Shark cartilage is an ideal, basic holistic supplement for bones and joint to which can be added a number of other natural agents to enhance its benefits (Table 1).

The value of cartilage supplements was recognized by several nutraceutical companies in the early 1990's. These companies started to look at individual components of cartilage and extract them as fractions for use alone or in simple combinations. The two components of cartilage supplements that attracted most interest were glucosamine-like compounds (GAG) and chondroitins. A focus of these components of cartilage is the basis of Cosequin® (a product sold by Nutramax Labs) and other popular nutraceuticals for joint health. These simple combinations of nutraceuticals are somewhat "passé", given more recent nutraceutical advances.

The popularization of simply combining glucosamine and chondroitin in a nutraceutical occurred largely as a consequence of the publication of the book "The Arthritis Cure" by Jason Theodosakis, Brenda Adderly and Barry Fox (St. Martin's Press, NY, NY, 1997). This book had a misleading name and advertised a "cure" for osteoarthritis, but no such cure exists! There is an impressive body of medical literature that supports the benefit of glucosamine and or chondroitin in osteoarthritis, with measurable benefits in terms of cartilage repair, renewal and regeneration in damaged joints. Whilst glucosamine and chondroitin use are real advances, the term "cure" is an overstatement, when applied to these nutraceuticals.

Modern nutritional science has recognized with clarity the advantage of glucosamine and chondroitin for joint health (Table 6), but these agents are present to all intents and purposes in cartilage supplements. It seems strange that "marketing hype" was able to push healthcare consumers to use extracts of cartilage when cartilage is "in itself" a much more complete (holistic) supplement than glucosamine alone or in combination with chondroitin. In addition, shark cartilage contains calcium, phosphorus, type II collagen, trace minerals and patented antiangiogenic proteins that are not present in glucosamine/chondroitin supplements and many of their variants. Chondroitin that is present in many glucosamine/chondroitin mixes is of bovine (cow) origin. This has led to major concerns about the transfer among species of Transmissible Spongiform Encephalopathy (TSE or mad cow disease). Chondroitin of bovine origin from Europe must be considered suspect. This problem does not present itself with shark cartilage.

In order to promote one brand or variant of glucosamine supplements over another, manufacturers have started to compare physical characteristics and types of glucosamine. In general, it is safe to say that all high quality glucosamine additions to joint supplements are valuable for bone and joint health (Table 6). There is little if any evidence that one well prepared type of glucosamine is better than the other and the arguments of the benefits of glucosamine sulphate versus chloride or vice versa do not "hold water", i.e. they are not tenable arguments. We cannot see the reason for "all the fuss" when extracts of cartilage, which were known to benefit arthritis, became down staged by glucosamine and chondroitin alone or in combination (these are essentially extracts of whole cartilage, or related components of shellfish in the case of glucosamine).

Davidson G. Glucosamine and Chondroitin Sulfate Pharm Profile. Compendium
    22(5):454-458 (2000)
Anderson MA: Oral chondroprotective agents. Part II. Evaluation of products.
    Compendium on Continuing Education for the Practicing Veterinarian
    21(9):861-865, 1999.
Anderson MA: Oral chondroprotective agents. Part 1. Common compounds.
    Compendium on Continuing Education for the Practicing Veterinarian
    21(7):601-609, 1999.
McAlindon T, La Valley M, Gulin J, Felson D, Glucosamine and Chondroitin for
    Treatment of Osteoarthritis JAMA 283:11 1469-1475, March 15, 2000.
Hanson RR: Oral glycosaminoglycans in the treatment of degenerative joint dis-
    ease in horses. Equine Practice 18(10):18-22, 1996.
Davis WM: The role of glucosamine and chondroitin sulfate in the management
    of arthritis. Drug Topics (Supplement):3S-13S, April 1998.
Hungerford DS: Treating osteoarthritis with chondroprotective agents. Orthopedic
    Special Edition 4(1):39-42, 1998.
Das A: The biochemistry of cartilage and osteoarthritis treatment options. A CME
    Accredited Special Report. New York, McMahon Publishing Group, pp
    1-4, January 1999.
Hulse DS: Treatment methods for pain in the osteoarthritic patient. The
    Veterinary Clincis of North America: Small Animal Practice 28(2):361,
    1998.
Schenck RC: Osteoarthritis treatment and potential structure modification with
    nutraceuticals. A CME Accredited Special Report. New York, McMahon
    Publishing Group, pp 1-4, August 1999.
Hungerford D, Navarro R, Hammad T: Use of nutraceuticals in the management
    of osteoarthritis. Journal of the American Nutraceutical Association
    3(1):23-27, 2000.
McLaughlin R: Management of chronic osteoarthritic pain. The Veterinary Clinics
    of North America: Small Animal Practice 30(4):939-943, 2000.
McNamara PS, Johnson SA, Todhunter RJ: Slow-acting disease-modifying
    osteoarthritis agents. The Veterinary Clinics of North America, Small
    Animal Practice 27(4):863-867, 951-952, 1997.
Lippiello L, Idouraine A, McNamara PS, Barr SC, McLaughlin RM. Cartilage
    Stimulatory and Antiproteolytic Activity is Present in Sera of Dogs
    Treated with a Chondroprotective Agent, Canine Practice, 24(1):18-19,
    January-February 1999.

Table 6

Some key recent articles that have been published on extracts of cartilage (chondroitin) and glucosamine. For further references see "The Arthritis Cure" by
J. Theodosakis MD et al and The Arthritis Solution by S. Messonier DVM.

It is clear that cartilage supplements and glucosamine plus or minus chondroitin have been superseded by more complex formulations of nutraceutical products for bone and joint health (Table 1 and Table 3). Whilst manufacturers argue that adding trace elements e.g. magnesium to glucosamine is beneficial, cartilage supplements do contain a wide array of natural minerals of marine origin. Nutraceutical technology for bone and joint health has graduated beyond simple cartilage supplements (e.g. shark cartilage) and simple combination products of glucosamine, chondroitin and minerals (e.g. Cosequin). This graduation in nutraceutical science has led to the development of new holistic bone and joint formulae to provide nutritional support. (Table 3).

The Synergy of New, Dynamic, Innovative Nutraceuticals for Bone and Joint Health: The PLUS factor

This discussion has focused on osteoarthritis (OA), the commonest form of arthritis encountered in dogs, cats and horses. Because OA is primarily a disease of cartilage, modern science has directed its attention to the use of compounds that protect cartilage. This protection is reflected in the term "chondroprotection", where "chondro" means "cartilage" that can be protected. Glucosamine, chondroitin and cartilage supplements are examples of "chondroprotective nutraceuticals". Chondroprotection is believed to be a more rational approach to dealing with OA in holistic care, than suppression of inflammation with NSAID or corticosteroids.

Dr. Shawn Messonier DVM, in his excellent book "The Arthritis Solution" has drawn attention to the advantages of using several different types of complementary therapies that "can be used simultaneously in an effort to maximize the chance of successful outcome". The combined approach promoted by Dr. Messonier and others is consistent with the use of a combination of synergistic nutraceuticals (Table 3). Synergy in formulation is the practice of mixing agents to get an additive effect that is greater than the use of single or simple combinations alone. These concepts are the "advanced" components of modern nutraceutical technology that have been used to develop new holistic bone and joint formulae.

Earlier in this section, we summarized many of the more popular nutraceuticals that have a credible basis for use in the support of bone and joint health (Table 1). Combining those nutraceuticals with a rational basis for enhancing joint mobility, protecting cartilage and combating joint problems is the basis of the formulation of new complete and holistic formulae for bone and joint health in pets (Table 3). The underlying principles and science behind the formulation of these formulae requires some scrutiny.

The Components of holistic Bone and Joint Formulae

The fundamental basis of the holistic formulae for bone and joint health is built around the basic benefits of cartilage supplements (shark cartilage researched as Cartilade in humans, CartiVet in dogs and cats and Cartequine in horses). Added to this base are extra glucosamine, hydrolyzed collagen, methylsulphonylmethane, Boswellia serrata, bromelain (enzymes), New Zealand Green Lipped Mussel, Brewers yeast and vitamin C (Table 3). Each of these ingredients has a well-defined role in musculoskeletal health that can be analyzed on an individual basis.

Hydrolyzed Type II Collagen

The story of the intriguing benefits of type II collagen (hydrolyzed collagen) in the treatment of arthritis came from research performed mainly by veterinary scientists. Therefore, it is quite surprising that this natural approach with collagen supplements has received more clinical research interest and treatment application in human medicine.

Both cartilage and protein hydrolysates of cartilage (protein partially broken down into its component amino acids) have been investigated as possible "chondroprotectants". Some of these preparations are enriched with amino acids such as L-cysteine. Protein hydrolysates that have been obtained mostly from collagen of animal origin contain a characteristic array of amino acids, most notably hydroxyproline, glycine, and hydroxylysine. These amino acids play a major role as building blocks for cartilage repair and nourishment and they are necessary for the biosynthesis of collagen.

Significant evidence has emerged that regular oral intake of protein hydrolysates of animal origin may stimulate hair or nail growth and skin health. It is frequently reported by patients or pet owner's that the taking of shark cartilage results in better hair growth, and trainers of horses and dogs have remarked on improvements in the skin and coats of these animals. This is not surprising, considering the similar embryological origins of these tissues. Furthermore, empirical (laboratory) and limited clinical studies have shown that animal protein hydrolysate-containing products may play a beneficial role in arthritis therapy, with both a pain reducing and "supportive role" in improving mobility. However, hydrolysates alone do not contain the entire spectrum of nutrients found in 100% pure shark cartilage.

Professor M. Adam of the Rheumaforschung Institute in Prague, Czech Republic, undertook a double-blind controlled trial (the type trial approved by conventional medicine) of 52 patients with significant, symptomatic osteoarthritis, who were given protein hydrolysate derived from bovine collagen and cartilage. The patients were split into groups and received purified protein hydrolysates or an active compound (drug). With the use of pure protein hydrolysates over a two-month period, improvements in symptoms of arthritis and decrease in analgesic (painkiller) consumption were noted.

Understanding Collagen's Role: Professor Norman Staines Hits the Mark !

Professor Norman Staines and his colleagues at King's College Medical School in London have performed excellent work on the role of collagen in the induction and treatment of experimentally induced arthritis in animals (Staines et al., 1990). Both articular and hyaline cartilage contain several types of genetically distinct collagens, of which Type II (C II) is the most common. Type II collagen can be solubilized by enzymes that break up the proteins into chains of amino acids (a process called proteolysis or artificial digestion).

This soluble derivative of native C II collagen can induce arthritis when injected into a rat, mouse, or primate. This collagen-induced arthritis in animals bears considerable resemblance to the disease of rheumatoid arthritis in humans. In addition, the immunological mechanisms of collagen-induced arthritis appear similar to those in human rheumatoid disease. Collagen-induced arthritis may often resolve spontaneously to a variable degree, just like it does in humans and animals. The work of Professor Staines and his group has been underemphasized in its importance. This research has been lost in the basic science literature.

Professor Staines and his colleagues gave injections of hydrolysates of bovine cartilage (containing "foreign" Type II collagen) to rats. When a rat receives this foreign collagen in its body, its immune system mounts an immune response. The rat has cartilage of its own, and with injections of foreign collagen, antibodies and other immune mechanisms kick into gear to attack the cartilage that is in the joints of the rats. The rat invariably develops an inflammatory (immune) arthritis as a consequence of receiving the injections of cartilage. This is an "autoimmune" triggering of the rat's arthritis, resembling human rheumatoid arthritis, causing a disease that resembles human rheumatoid arthritis. Now, here is the magic of the observations. If the rat is fed (by mouth) the cartilage products, the rat is often protected against the development of the immune-mediated, inflammatory arthritis that was induced by the injection of the foreign cartilage.

The Hypothesis: How Cartilage and its Collagen May Work in Arthritis

The mechanism whereby the oral feeding of foreign cartilage protects against the development of immune, inflammatory arthritis in animals is related to the induction of what is called "immune tolerance". This means that feeding the cartilage extracts that have also been injected results in a state of tolerance in the experimental animal. The immune system of the rat will not be triggered to attack its own joints. Immune tolerance induced by oral cartilage stops the self-destruction of the joints by the rat's own immune system.

It has been postulated that bits of cartilage or compounds from cartilage can enter the circulation of a human or animal and trigger an immune response. In simple terms: If a bit of cartilage from an individual's own joint triggers that person's own immune system to attack their own joints, then an inflammatory arthritis will occur. We know that cartilage is found in an " immunologically privileged site". The means that the body's immune system does not readily get to meet or recognize cartilage in normal joints, so it does not normally make an immune attack. If a joint is injured, stressed, infected, or damaged, the cartilage is exposed to the immune system and an immune response will cause arthritis. Here is the "ringer". Oral cartilage supplements may induce the immune tolerance phenomenon in humans and pets in the same way that oral cartilage induced the immune tolerance phenomenon in the rats that were injected with collagen in order to induce an immune, inflammatory arthritis. This important research work prompted the inclusion of hydrolyzed collagen in new holistic bone and joint food supplements (Table 3).

Vitamin C

The failure to include vitamin C in many bone and joint supplements for pets is a serious omission. Vitamin C has been shown to play a special treatment role in dysplasia (abnormal growth and development of joints), especially hip dysplasia in dogs. Vitamin C is a classic antioxidant. One reads a great deal about the health benefits of antioxidants, which prevent "oxidative damage" to tissues. Oxidative damage to tissues is very important in almost every chronic disease including diseases of joints, glands, the heart and the immune system. Antioxidants, like vitamin C, neutralize reactive oxygen molecules or "free radicals" and prevent oxidative damage to tissues.

According to several holistic vets, Vitamin C and other antioxidants may be quite helpful in pain relief and reduction of inflammation in stressed, injured or arthritic joints. Furthermore, evidence has accumulated that vitamin C may actually prevent arthritis and bone and joint problems, such as hip dysplasia. Dr. Shawn Messonier DVM draws attention to the importance of vitamin C for joint health in his book "The Arthritis Solution".

The issues concerning the benefits of vitamin C are clouded by the knowledge that dogs can manufacture vitamin C for themselves. Some individuals have argued against the occurrence of deficiency states. However, very impressive research by Dr. Wendell O. Belfield DVM suggests that vitamin C can be given to pets to both prevent and treat hip dysplasia and other types of arthritis. Dr. Belfield went further in his research conclusions and proposed that

vitamin C can actually assist in cases of osteochondrosis and gener-
alized osteoarthritis. Dr. Belfield has reported his research in the
classic textbook "Complementary and Alternative Veterinary
Medicine: Principles and Practice (Edited by AM Schoen DVM and
Susan G Wynn DVM).

In brief, Dr. Belfield studied eight litters of German Shepherd
pups who were derived from a family line of dogs that had a strong
history of hip dysplasia. In classic, veterinary, medical literature, hip
dysplasia has been considered to be primarily a birth defect (genetic
or inherited disorder). In Dr. Belfield's study of German Shepherd
dogs with a tendency to dysplasia of the hips, the administration of
vitamin C in pregnancy resulted in no signs of hip dysplasia in the
offspring.

Whilst Dr. Belfield's study has been debated, there are good
reasons to believe that vitamin C may be beneficial for normal functions of muscles, bones and joints. Vitamin C is absolutely necessary for the optimal development of muscles, bones, cartilage and
their attachments. Conventional approaches to the prevention or
treatment of hip dysplasia include selective breeding, conservative
therapy, drugs and complex surgery. All of these orthodox approaches
possess disadvantages and limitations.

Whilst more research is required in this area, the idea that hip
dysplasia and other musculoskeletal problems may be controlled by
vitamin C is intriguing. For these reasons, complete bone and joint
supplements contain a generous supply of vitamin C that is often
missing in some food supplements.

New Zealand Green-Lipped Mussel (Perna canaliculus)

Marine life provides a variety of components of highly beneficial nutraceuticals. Glucosamine is extracted from shellfish and it
is one example of a group of substances called glycoaminoglycans
(GAG). We learned that these molecules (GAG) are present in cartilage supplements and much evidence exists for their benefits as
natural anti-inflammatory agents that provide chondroprotection.
The green-lipped mussel from New Zealand is an especially good
source of GAG and certain types of chondroitin. It is the GAG,
chondroitin and trace mineral content of the green-lipped mussel

that makes it a valuable nutraceutical for bone and joint function.

Derivatives of green-lipped mussel have been found to be very valuable in the management of osteoarthritis and hip dysplasia. They are believed to contribute to pain reduction and enhanced mobility in dogs, cats and horses. Clinical trials suggest a credible benefit of green-lipped mussel in osteoarthritis and it works very well in combination with glucosamine and methylsulfonylmethone (MSM). Combination products have appeared with green-lipped mussel but none are complete (Table 3).

MSM - Methylsulfonylmethane

MSM has been described as a highly effective anti-inflammatory agent with pain relieving properties. It has found a special role for inclusion in bone and joint, dietary supplements for humans and it is being applied increasingly in veterinary practice. Whilst it is effective for joint disorders, it is an ideal companion ingredient, rather than a "stand-alone", joint supplement. MSM is derived from DMSO (dimethylsulfoxide), which has been used as a carrier substance and "topical rub" for bone and joint problems in pets, especially horses. DMSO itself has some problems, even though it has been widely used.

MSM works by supplying the element sulfur to the body. Sulfur is a very important substance that is essential for the growth and nourishment of cartilage and connective tissues. Books have been written about the health benefit of MSM but they have tended to oversensationalize its use by using words like "miracles". There is a body of opinion among food scientists that pets (and human) diets may be often deficient in sulfur. Although several foods contain MSM, it can be lost in cooking or food storage.

Dr. Shawn Messonier DVM has discussed studies of the composition of cartilage in arthritic joints, where the concentration of sulfur in damaged cartilage may be grossly reduced. Several clinical trials in humans and animals have shown that MSM can effectively reduce pain, improve joint mobility, enhance joint flexibility and exert anti-inflammatory effects. One striking observation that deserves further research is the apparent ability of MSM to prevent cartilage damage in inflammatory types of arthritis, such as rheumatoid disease.

MSM appears to be quite safe unless used in very high doses for prolonged periods of time. No side effects have been seen in humans given MSM for several months. In modest doses MSM is an ideal synergistic addition to a bone and joint nutraceutical (Table 3).

Boswellia serrata

Boswellia is extracted from gum resins derived from the tree Boswellia serrata. The extract belongs to a class of compounds called gugguls, which have been described in ancient Ayurvedic medicine as possessing potent, antirheumatic properties. Ayurvedic medicine is a complex medical philosophy that was developed a couple of thousand years ago on the Indian subcontinent. It uses special lifestyle approaches and a variety of herbal or botanical remedies. The active ingredients of boswellia extracts are beta-boswellic acid and other related acids.

Many studies have confirmed the benefit of standardized boswellia extract in the treatment of osteoarthritis and rheumatoid arthritis. Boswellic acids can protect against artificially induced arthritis in animals and the herb's anti-inflammatory actions have been well documented in soft tissue inflammation. Detailed laboratory experiments have shown that extracts of Boswellia serrata resins protect the main constituents of bone and cartilage by reducing the activity of several enzymes that degrade important structural components of cartilage (glycosaminoglycans).

Some scientists have referred to Boswellia as a natural, non-steroidal anti-inflammatory agent. This suggestion is not to be confused with standard non-steroidal anti-inflammatory drugs (NSAID's), such as carprofen, etodolac, meclofenamic acid and phenylbutazone (Bute), which often produce stomach or duodenal ulcers. It is notable that Boswellia exhibits antiulcerogenic activity, in contrast to the ulcerogenic (ulcer causing) potential of NSAID. The NSAID (e.g. carprofen, etodolac, meclofenamic acid) inhibit cyclooxygenase enzymes, whereas Boswellia inhibits enzymes that form leukotrienes (substances that provoke inflammation).

Dietary supplements containing standardized extracts of Boswellia have been reported repeatedly to reduce joint swelling and morning stiffness, increase joint mobility, and produce an overall improvement in quality of life in arthritic subjects. These effects have been seen in patients with a variety of rheumatological disorders such as: osteoarthritis, gouty arthritis, rheumatoid disease, nonspecific rheumatism, fibrositis, myositis, cervical spondylolysis, and backache due to vertebral disorders. Boswellia is finding an increasing role as a dietary supplement in the treatment of arthritis in humans, dogs with hip dysplasia, and lame horses.

Bromelain

Bromelain is a mixture of certain, protein-digesting enzymes (proteolytic enzymes) that are found in the stems of pineapples. Most bromelain is contained in the stem of the pineapple nearest to the fruit. Concentrations of bromelain are also found in the woody core of pineapples.

There are more than one hundred scientific studies supporting the use of bromelain as potential therapy for arthritis, sports injuries, and soft tissue trauma. Bromelain has anti-inflammatory effects, including some demonstrated ability to block the production of compounds that mediate inflammation. Bromelain is a valuable component of dietary supplements used to promote joint health, and the supporting evidence for this application is strong. Bromelain is very useful for taking care of the soft tissue problems that occur around joints that are stressed or arthritic. This enzyme preparation from pineapples is quite valuable in the control of "shin splints" and strains in competitive horses and dogs. Many bone and joint health products are devoid of nutraceutical components to take care of the inevitable soft tissue problems in active pets (Table 3).

Brewer's Yeast

Whilst scientists may obsess about the actions of specific nutraceuticals, they may tend to forget the holistic, health-giving properties of "age-old" food components such as common yeasts. Dried yeasts are a veritable powerhouse of health-giving nutrients and they have well defined nutraceutical, treatment benefits in a variety of circumstances. It is easy to underestimate the nutritional force of Brewer's yeast, but its attraction to dogs, cats and horses is obvious - they love its taste! It is the nutritional value and palatability of Brewer's yeast that makes it so attractive as a supplement in our pets' diets.

The first myth to dispel is that yeast has anything to do with yeast infections due to the organism Candida albicans that causes "thrush" or Candidiasis. Brewer's yeast and dried yeast are not capable of causing any infections. They are prepared by special drying procedures that make their nutritional components readily available for digestion into the body of a pet. Brewer's yeast is a single-celled plant called Saccharomyces cerevisiae. As it grows, it develops an excellent content of protein (composed of essential amino acids), vitamins (especially B complex), essential minerals and other health-giving substances.

The approximate analysis of Brewer's yeast is shown in Table 7. The nutritive composition of yeast is so varied and complete that it shocks many people when they see its nutritional components for the first time. One important fact that is well documented in nutritional science is that Brewer's yeast has a nutritional value to an animal or human that exceeds that of mixtures of the recognized (known) components that are present in the dried plant (yeast). In other terms, giving the known constituents of yeast in mixtures does not result in all of the nutritional benefits that are encountered by giving whole Brewer's yeast.

BREWER'S YEAST HAS NOTHING TO DO WITH YEAST INFECTIONS (CANDIDA). IT IS A POWERHOUSE OF VITAL NUTRIENTS.

Approximate analysis		Vitamin Potencies (micrograms per gram)	
Protein	50.0%	Thiamine (B1)	150
Purine Nitrogen	0.4%	Riboflavin (B2)	50
Total Carbohydrates	31.7%	Niacin	400
Fat (ether extractable)	1.2%	Pyridoxine (B6)	40
Total Lipids	5.8%	Pantothenic Acid	100
Moisture	5.0%	Biotin	1.25
Calories (per gram)	3.5	Choline	3350
Ash	7.5%	Inositol	4425
		Folic acid	5
Calcium	0.125%		
Phosphorus	1.5%		
Potassium	1.62%		
Magnesium	0.25%		
Sodium	0.22%		
Copper	8.5 ppm		
Iron	55.0 ppm		
Zinc	45.0 ppm		
Manganese	6.5 ppm		

Table 7

Brewer's yeast, dried yeast. These are approximate values that vary by preparation methods. Data taken from yeast manufacturer's information.

Brewer's yeast is a source of high quality protein, which contains several essential amino acids (Table 8). Whilst yeast is low in its content of the amino acid methionine, this amino acid is abundant in most pets' diets. The carbohydrate and fat content of Brewer's yeast is desirably low. Its content of "neutral fats" gives it antioxidant properties.

Amino Acids	Percent in Dried Yeast Protein	Daily for Nitrogen Balance in Adult Man
Arginine	4.7	—
Aspartic acid	8.2	—
Cystine	0.9	—
Glutamic acid	15.3	—
Glycine	3.7	—
Histidine	1.5	—
Isoleucine	5.7	0.7
Leucine	6.3	1.1
Lysine	7.3	0.8
Methionine	1.2	1.1
Phenylatanine	4.4	1.1
Serine	3.9	—
Threonine	4.8	0.5
Tryptophan	1.1	0.25
Tyrosine	3.4	—
Valine	5.2	0.8

Table 8

Amino acid content of Brewer's Yeast. Approximate values taken from data produced by yeast manufacturers.

The mineral content of Brewer's yeast is especially valuable. It contains calcium and phosphorus to help good bone formation, iron for red blood cell formation and selenium, a powerful antioxidant. Selenium deficiency in pets' diets has been regarded as a particular problem that is deserving of frequent correction. Brewer's yeast is best known for its very good profile of vitamins of the B complex. Dried yeast contains more than ten separate vitamin B complex components including: thiamine, riboflavin, niacin, pyridoxine, pantothenic acid, biotin, choline, inositol, folic acid and paraminobenzoic acid (PABA). The vitamin B complex has many vital functions in the body of humans and animals.

In addition, to the nutrient content of Brewer's yeast, there are several other substances present that have been called "dietary protective factors" in yeast. One such factor is called Factor 3 that contains selenium and another is "glucose tolerance factor" which contains chromium. These factors have wide-ranging health potential in terms of antioxidant actions and blood glucose control, respectively.

A very novel aspect of Brewer's yeast is its ability to stimulate immune function. This property is related to the content of a special, big sugar (polysaccharide) called beta glucan. Much recent literature has focused on the ability of beta glucan from yeast to stimulate white cells in the immune system and balance other aspects of immunity.

In summary, Brewer's yeast is one of the most versatile and potent, natural "nutraceuticals" with wide ranging health potential. It may be more than a coincidence that pets love Brewer's yeast. Perhaps this is a special trick of nature!

The formulation and use of Holistic Bone and Joint Formulae

The formulation of nutraceuticals for bone and joint health has evolved from ten years of research and development in nutraceuticals (Table 3). Major advances have been made with the use of natural agents (herbs, botanicals and nutrients) for the support of bone and joint structure and function. The complete nature of the ingredients found in Table 3 make it the quintessential currentbone and joint supplement.

Holistic bone and joint formulae should contain glucosamine, hydrolyzed collagen, MSM, Boswellia serrata, vitamin C, New Zealand Green Lipped mussel and Brewer's yeast in the holistic base of patented shark cartilage. Each of the components of any formulae should have a significant amount of research to support its use for bone and joint health. In some cases, the natural ingredients recommended have been shown to be effective in controlled clinical trials. These products should be formulated to veterinarian, clinical grade and contain bioactive nutraceuticals that work in an additive manner (synergism).

As dietary supplements, the ingredients of proposed holistic bone and joint food supplemenrs work together to:

1. **Provide chondroprotection (protect cartilage in joints)**
2. **Exert anti-inflammatory effects**
3. **Provide nutrient building blocks for bones and joints**
4. **Assist in the repair, renewal and regeneration of cartilage**
5. **Bromelain helps deal with soft tissue problems around joints**
6. **Improve pain and joint mobility**
7. **Provide an array of vitamins and minerals to support several body functions and structures**
8. **Provide natural agents that support immune function e.g. vitamin C, beta glucan in yeast**
9. **Provide antioxidant action**
10. **Provide antiangiogenic proteins and interference with unwanted leukotriene synthesis (Boswellia).**

Holistic nutraceutical combinations with wide ranging benefits for the support of musculoskeletal structure and function in pets (cats, dogs and horses) now exist. Our proposals are more complete in their contents than other, popular bone and joint supplements as illustrated by a comparison of its composition in Table 9.

Holistic PLUS formulae

Cosequin—Glycoflex—Arthriease V-P—Arthri-Nu—Flexagan II—HipHealth—PLUS™—PLUS™

	Cosequin	Glycoflex	Arthriease V-P	Arthri-Nu	Flexagan II	HipHealth	PLUS™	PLUS™
Substantial calcium and phosphate content	-	-	-	-	-	-	X	x
Glucosmaine	-	X	X	X	-	X	X	x
Chondroitin	-	-	X	-	-	-	X	x
Hydrolyzed collagen	X	-	-	-	-	-	X	x
MSM	X	-	-	-	X	-	X	x
Boswellia	X	-	X	-	-	-	X	x
Essential trace minerals	X	X	X	X	-	X	X	x
Bromelain	-	-	-	-	-	X	X	x
Green Lipped Mussel	-	X	-	-	-	-	X	x
Vitamin C	-	-	-	-	-	X	X	x
Patented Antiangiogenic ingredient	-	x	x	-	-	-	X	X
	-	-	-	-	-	-	X	X
General immune boost Beta glucan	-	x	x	-	-	-	X	X

Table 9

Plus formulae are the most complete, natural, bone and joint health products. It has the widest range of synergistic nutraceutical components to support joint structure and function. Comparison of bone and joint products for animals. (Reproduced with permission of Natures Benefit, Inc.)

Summary

Table 10 provides a list of conventional food supplement treatment options. Among nutraceuticals, CartiVet Plus™ and Cartequine Plus™ are complete.

Trade Name	Available Form	Composition
Arthramine	Tablets	Glucosamine
		Vitamins
		Bromelain
		Feverfew
		Manganese
ArthriEase V-P	Powder	Glucosamine
		Vitamins
		Antioxidants
		Yucca
		Boswellin
		Chondroitin Sulfate
Arthri-nu	Powder	Glucosamine
		Antioxidants
Arthroflex	Powder	Glycosaminoglycans
Best Hip and joint	Tablets	Glucosamine
		Antioxidants
		Boswellin
		Yucca
		Minerals
Cartiflex	Capsules	Glycosaminoglycans
CartiVet PLUS	Powder	Glucosamine
		Hydrolyzed Collagen
		MSM
		Calcium
		Phosphorus
		Brewers Yeast
		Trace elements
		Perna Canaliculus
		Boswellia
		Bromelain
		Shark Cartilage
		(Chondroitin types A&C)
		Vitamin C

Cartequine PLUS	Powder	see CartiVet PLUS
Cosequine	Capsules	Glucosamine
		Chondroitin Sulfate
Flexagan II	Tablets	MSM
Glucosmeg	Liquid, Tablets	Glucosamine
		Vitamins
GlycoFlex	Tablets	Glycosaminoglycans
		Chelated Minerals
		Vitamins
		Enzymes
		Amino Acids
		Nucleic Acids
GlycoFlex Plus	Tablets	Glycosaminoglycans
		Chelated Minerals
		Vitamins
		Enzymes
		Amino Acids
		Nucleic Acids
		MSM
Hip Health	Powder	Glucosamine
		Vitamins
		Amino Acids
Synovi-care	Tablets	Glucosamine
		Glycosaminoglycans
		Creatine
		Amono Acids
		Antioxidants
Synovi-MSM	Powder	Glucosamine
		MSM
		Perna Canliculus
		Vitamin C

NSAID	Side Effects	Dosage
Aspirin	Gastric ulceration, anemia	10-25 mg/kg orally 2-3 times daily
Rimadyl (Carprofen)	Gastrointestinal, renal and hepatic disorders and	2.2 mg/kg orally every 12 hours
EtoGesic (Etodolac)	lethargy, vomiting, diarrhea	10-15 mg/kg every 24 hours
Arquel (Meclofenamic Acid)	diarrhea, renal compromise and death	1.1 mg/kg orally divided into 2-3 doses daily
Phenylbutazone	Hepatitis, GI injury, nephropathy and death	8-16 mg/kg orally 2 times daily

Surgical Options

Arthrodesis, Arthroscopic Debridement, Excision Arthroplasty, Synovectomy, Total Joint Replacement	Discuss all of these option with veterinary surgeon

Table 10
A list of conventional and natural treatments for bone and joint health.

The National Bone Disease Survey of Linda Arndt

There have been numerous arguments about the causation of bone and joint problems in companion animals. Linda Arndt is an expert breeder of Great Danes and she has made one of the most important contributions to our understanding of bone and joint problems in dogs. She undertook a mammoth survey of skeletal problems in Great Danes and showed unequivocal evidence that most bone and joint problems are caused by poor nutrition. Whilst increasing numbers of informed pet owners have accepted the importance of nutrition in the maintenance of skeletal health, a substantial proportion of practicing veterinarians have not embraced nutritional theories for bone and joint health. This is not surprising given the focus of conventional medical practices on drug therapies and surgery. In fact, the same situation exists in human medicine where allopathic physicians have been very slow to use nutritional therapies for bone and joint health.

This fixation with drugs is surprising, because anti-arthritis drugs, such as non-steroidal anti-inflammatory drugs, are so often associated with severe side effects and sometimes death. Established or progressive arthritis rarely presents an acute medical emergency and it seems inappropriate to rush to prescription drug therapy, with its known risks, without exercising simple and gentle natural options. Linda Arndt's work is so important that we asked her permission to report some of her findings in detail. For individuals with a greater interest in this information Linda Arndt can be emailed at GrDaneLady@aol.com. Whilst Linda's work was with the large breed of Great Danes, her findings are very relevant to all companion animals. We have no reason to suspect that circumstances differ greatly in other breeds of dogs or even in cats.

The Survey

After many years of dedicated service to pet owners, Linda Arndt became very concerned about the common occurrence of bone and joint problems in Great Danes. In 1988, Linda started a prospective (forward looking) survey that ran for 5 years and involved a study of 5237 cases of bone and joint problems in Great Danes. Linda analyzed a vast amount of information and concluded that bone and joint problems were related to poor nutritional practices. These conclusions led her to recommend certain specific types of feeding practices to verify her conclusions. These feed trials involved 40 litters of Great Danes of all colors and bloodlines. Linda Arndt went as far as providing resources for veterinarian-based diagnosis of bone and joint disease, to provide objective scientific information.

Linda focused on three different types of disease affecting the skeletal structures of Great Danes. These diseases included Hypertrophic Osteodystrophy (HOD), Osteochrondritis Dissecans (OCD) and Panosteitis (Pano). Her detailed observations of these disorders permitted her to write a celebrated article entitled: "A Guide To Recognizing Bone Diseases", which was published in the Great Dane Reporter and several other large-dog breed magazines. One striking observation was the ability of allergic reactions to drugs (e.g. antibiotics) and vaccine responses to mimic these diseases. Out of much complex data, Linda was able to show that excessive calorie intake with unbalanced, common dog foods and lack of sufficient intake or balance of minerals (e.g. calcium, phosphorus and trace elements) caused joint diseases. In the case of Pano, calcium and phosphorus balance appeared to be particularly important. Linda demonstrated that poor nutrition, related to the composition of many commercial brands of dog food resulted in uneven growth patterns in dogs that were not easily reversible.

The Solution?

In common with Linda's conclusions, many nutritionists have stressed the importance of diet in the promotion of healthy bone and joint function. New attempts are being made to produce foods with a special health purpose for animals, but the formulation of many of these foods is inadequate and they are very expensive. Without more acknowledgement of the role of diet in companion animal well-being, the most effective route to correcting nutritional problems is to use dietary supplements in a prudent and judicious manner. Linda Arndt shares the opinion of many concerned pet owners and breeders who are increasingly selecting specific supplements to correct nutritional imbalances that are created by popular commercial diets. At present, we do not have ideal functional foods for our pets, but we have many valuable natural supplements.

Natural agents for joint pain and mobility: the story of cyclooxygenase inhibition

Fifty five million Americans (one quarter of the population) have significant arthritis and every adult at some stage in their life requires relief of musculoskeletal pain. Arthritis, stress injury and related conditions are even more common proportionately in cats, dogs and horses. The conventional treatment of bone and joint disorders has been most often achieved by the use of aspirin, acetaminophen and a host of non-steroidal, anti-inflammatory drugs (NSAID) in humans. However, NSAID have been described as a major public health concern, as a consequence of their common, multiple and onerous side effects; which include: dyspepsia, peptic ulceration, bleeding diatheses, renal insufficiency and liver impairment. The use of NSAID in companion animals presents similar problems. When it comes to popular NSAID used in animals e.g. Rimadyl (Carprofen), EtoGesic (Etodolac), Arquel (Meclofenamic Acid) and Phenylbutazone, the same serious and sometimes fatal side effects occur, as they do in humans. Much media attention has focused on deaths in dogs from the use of Carprofen.

The NSAID work by inhibiting an enzyme system called cyclooxygenase (COX). This enzymes system has been described as occurring in two basic forms, type I and type II. In simple terms these enzyme systems COX-1 and COX-2 cause inflammation to occur, especially in joints. Blocking these enzymes will diminish inflammation, but at the same time it will adversely affect some body functions or structures e.g. the lining of the gastrointestinal tract and the functions of the liver and kidneys. Recent promises that new types of NSAID that work only on COX-2 enzymes are much less damaging in side effects have not come true. Selective COX-2 inhibiting types of NSAID cause gastrointestinal, liver and kidney problems.

Warnings not heeded!

The medical literature of the past three decades is replete with warnings about the adverse effects of NSAID. In humans, they are associated with more than 60% of all life threatening bleeding from the upper digestive tract and they contribute to lower gastrointestinal bleeding. The morbidity and mortality from NSAID use is most apparent in the elderly - the principal target population for their use. Mature individuals invariably suffer from "thin bones and creaky joints". NSAID dangers are acutely apparent when one recognizes that they are the commonest reason for adverse, drug, side effect reporting to the FDA. Whilst NSAID can do exactly the same thing in companion animals, far less attention has been focused on these problems in veterinary practice, until recently.

Limitations of "improved" NSAID - COX-2 inhibitors

For two decades, the "me to" category of NSAID has seen new product introductions, which are variations on a standard pharmacological (drug) theme of cyclooxygenase (COX) inhibition. We have often been told that "NSAID-X" was safer or more effective than "NSAID-Y", but several studies have indicated that these assertions may be only flimsy claims of better treatment outcome among "regular", non-selective types of NSAID. COX catalyses prostaglandin production and it occurs in two isoforms, COX-1 and COX-2 (Fig.1). Traditional NSAID inhibit both isoforms of cyclooxygenase, whereas newer forms of NSAID (e.g. rofecoxib or celecoxib) more selectively inhibit COX-2. The notion that COX-1 plays an essential role in normal gut and platelet function and COX-2 is induced by inflammatory processes afforded medical practitioners a "new promise" for the enhanced safety, but not necessarily efficacy, of NSAID that work only on COX-2. The new promise has not been realized.

Until recently, the jury remained out on whether or not COX-2, NSAID are "friendly" to the gastrointestinal tract. They are not friendly and they cause ulcers and gastrointestinal bleeding. Recent studies confirm that COX-2 inhibition causes significant decreases in renal function, at least equivalent, if not greater than, regular NSAID. One may anticipate that liver impairment may occur in some patients taking COX-2 inhibition. Thus, the massive swing toward the human prescription use of COX-2, NSAID compared with regular NSAID (inhibition of COX-1 and COX-2) may not be as reassuring as hitherto supposed. As with all new classes of drugs, time will tell and there are a few, less well-known, worries about COX-2 inhibition (Fig. 1).

DIETARY SUPPLEMENTS CANNOT BE USED TO DIAGNOSE, PREVENT OR TREAT ANY DISEASE.

Arachidonic Acid
CONVERSION TO PROSTAGLANDINS

COX-1
(Constitutive gene)

COX-2
(Inducible gene)

Prostaglandins and
thromboxanes

Prostaglandins

- Promote mucosal integrity
  (especially the gut)
- Platelet aggregation
- Renal Function
- Selected CNS and liver function
- Selectivity? Note: nabumetone and
  etodolac are alleged preferential COX-2
  inhibitors. They result in GI toxicity.
- COX-2 selectively of all COX-2 inhibition
  NSAID may be lost at high doses! More
  about "me to", NSAID are emerging with
  properties - unnecessary?

- Induced role in inflammation
- Mitogenesis and
  growth (COX-2 inhibition
  useful in cancer therapy?)
- Regulation of reproduction
  in females (concerns of COX-2
  inhibition of ovulation, placental
  implantation, pregnancy, delays
  in labor?
- Bone formation (concerns
  COX-2 induced changes in func
  tion of combined COX-1 and
  COX-2 inhibitory of osteoblasts
  and osteoclasts)
- Renal function, COX-inhibition
  significantly decreases renal
  function COX-2 is protective to GI
  function, contrary to popular
  belief !
- COX-2 inhibition could interfere
  with healing in some inflamma
  tory processes?

Figure 1: Unresolved concerns about COX-2 inhibition.
Common concerns exist about COX-1 and COX-2 inhibition. Readers are referred to
the American Pharmaceutical Association's teaching document on COX-2 inhibition.
COX-2 inhibitors may have more potential problems than hitherto supposed, but one
might expect that they will be introduced into veterinary practice in the near future.

Natural COX-2 inhibitors

Inhibiting the enzyme COX-2 in a potent manner using a drug is clearly associated with unwanted side effects. However, there are a series of naturally occurring compounds found in herbs and botanicals that show an ability to inhibit COX-2 without the side effects experienced with COX-2 inhibitor drugs. Individuals who are interested in this novel approach are referred to the website www.naturalcox-2inhibitor.com. In brief, these natural agents include: Barberry Bark, Goldenthread, Feverfew, Ginger Root, Green Tea, Tulsi Leaves, Hops, Oregano, Rosemary Leaf, Scullcap, Turmeric, Nettle Leaves and Polygonum Cuspidatum. One interesting herb is Phellodendron amurense, which has been produced in an extract form with clear COX-2 inhibiting activity. The basis of this knowledge has resulted in the development of a dietary supplement which is a Natural COX-2 inhibitor. It is a proprietary blend of natural agents that have anti-inflammatory potential, pain relieving properties, and beneficial effects on soft tissues associated with joints. One may think that inhibiting COX-2 is a bad idea, given the outcome of some uses of COX-2 inhibitor drugs, but nature appears to provide a mechanism to inhibit COX-2 in a beneficial manner that is safe, effective and gentle. The reasons for this are not clear.

Doing away with NSAID?

So pernicious are the problems of NSAID usage and so common are bone and joint problems, that many consumers are seeking alternative, natural remedies. People with arthritis often self-medicate and, after all, the OTC availability of NSAID is in its old, "regular" format (non-specific COX-1 and COX-2 inhibition). The iatrogenic (medical practitioner induced) diseases caused by NSAID provide powerful stimuli for patients, physicians and pharmacists to avoid their use. The enigma remains, however, that NSAID are the most commonly used drugs of all pharmaceutical categories in humans and they are increasingly used in companion animals, especially dogs.

Can we do away with NSAD use?

We believe that we have some real options in natural therapies to at least reduce the need for NSAID and, on occasion, completely avoid their use. We have learned that there are several bone and joint nutritional supplements for which there is mounting evidence of efficacy and clear advantages in terms of safety, over NSAID usage. By now, human healthcare givers are tired of reading truncated overviews of the benefits of individual, dietary supplements for joint health, but veterinarians have not been exposed to the same consumer demand for alternatives to drug therapy of arthritis in companion animals. Whilst we have learned a great deal about the properties of natural therapies for arthritis and musculoskeletal injuries, accounts of the most effective way to use natural remedies have been lacking (the "therapeutics" or practical use of natural remedies).

Effective use of natural bone and joint therapies

With perhaps the exception of Ayurvedic tree resins (Boswellic acids and Guggulsterones), most orally administered natural remedies for joint disorders take "many days" (or sometimes weeks) to be completely effective. For example, the natural anti-inflammatory actions of glucosamine, chondroitin or the holistic mixture of shark cartilage (calcium, phosphorus, glucosamine-like molecules, type II collagen and antiangiogenic proteins) can take as long as twelve weeks before maximal benefits are achieved. The cartilage regenerative powers of glucosamine and shark cartilage take even longer. We want to emphasize that well-controlled experiments in dogs have shown that NSAID (indomethacin) can actually damage cartilage. This contrarian effect of NSAID is very worrying. On the one hand, NSAID suppress inflammation, whereas, on the other, they have a possibility of making the disease worse over time. The conventional physician may argue against this but the facts speak for themselves. No drug therapy to date has been shown to significantly alter the natural history (overall outcome) of the progression of arthritis. In contrast, we believe that nutritional approaches will both help prevent joint problems and alter their clinical course.

Controlled, comparative clinical studies of certain NSAID and glucosamine show that NSAID "win out" in terms of symptomatic relief early in treatment, but over "weeks" their benefits equilibrate with those of NSAID and even result, over time, in better treatment outcome with glucosamine! In fact, we know that certain NSAID may damage cartilage, whereas glucosamine and shark cartilage have cartilage regenerative powers. Cartilage renewal, repair and regeneration with some of the components of holistic supplements are possible.

Recognizing that the delayed effects of oral bone and joint supplements are a drawback, one has to deal with the interim course of arthritis (pain, stiffness and reduced mobility) during its initial management. There are two viable options. First, it is often best to introduce natural therapies and "tail off" NSAID slowly, while the benefits of effective supplements "kick in". The second option is to use an effective topical pain relieving gels or creams, initially or in a synchronous manner with the switch from NSAID to selected natural therapies. Several, highly effective topical pain relief products have been recently launched which contain the active pain relieving, constituent capsaicin (from pepper plants).

The Capsaicin Advantage

Much credible evidence exists that capsaicin can effectively block pain from arthritic joints, by specific inhibition of the actions of substance P. This substance is a principal neurotransmitter of pain from visceral and somatic sources. Capsaicin creams have over the counter drug label claims for pain relief, approved by NDC registrations (and the FDA). When applied topically, capsaicin can variably penetrate the skin and with repeated application, pain relief improves with a crescendo effect at about seven to ten days - another drawback of delayed effect. However, if the cutaneous delivery of capsaicin is facilitated by liposomes, a maximal effect can be sometimes achieved much quicker - in about 72 hours! Furthermore, in selected cases in clinical studies the application of topical capsaicin can alone reduce the need for NSAID dosages by a factor of up to 80%.

The addition of essential oils of menthol and camphor to liposome containing capsaicin creams further amplifies and accelerates analgesia. When applied topically, these essential oils cool the skin and have a local anesthetic effect because they are freely diffusible. An added advantage of their inclusion is that they lessen the "prickly" or minor burning sensation that is induced often by topical application of capsaicin.

Certain "soothing" elements have been added to these capsaicin creams including: shark cartilage (for its glucosamine and chondroitin content), glucosamine, aloe vera and even agents such as MSM. Whilst it is questionable if the topical application of macromolecular substances, such as glucosamine, could access the body when applied topically, some healthcare givers claim efficacy.

Conclusion

We cannot be too "cocky" about the putative safety, advantages of NSAID. Topical pain relief with containing capsaicin creams and the simultaneous use of oral bone and joint supplements, e.g. holistic "plus" formulae (whilst "tailing off NSAID) has obvious advantages. We have natural therapeutic gifts for bone and joint problems that are best applied with approaches that maximize their beneficial properties.

Skin and Coat Health

Vibrant Skin and Coat

Our pet shares our pride when their coat is healthy. They feel "proud". Skin and coat health is a reflection of total body health in companion animals. Disorders of the skin and coat are the commonest problems that face pet owners (Table 11). Signs of health in the skin often come from within the body. Therefore, concentration on the use of topical (surface) products for coat health is sometimes misguided. The skin and coat is the largest organ in the body of a pet and it receives daily insults from the environment. Like any other vital organ of the body, the skin needs nutrients and a friendly environment to maintain its health. Many veterinarians agree that the pivotal factor in skin and coat health is optimal nutrition.

Hot spots	Bare patches
Acne in cats	Dull coat
Chronic itching	Bumpy (papular) rashes
Eczema	Excessive shedding
Pet odors	Dandruff
Pigment changes	Matting and brittle fur

Table 11

Common skin conditions in pets. These conditions arise frequently from poor nutrition, general ill health and sometimes "owner neglect".

Vital Nutrients for Skin Health

There are many nutrients that are required for optimal skin and fur conditioning. Animals that have irritated or inflamed skin disorders often benefit from a "modified fast". Giving the digestive tract a rest whilst maintaining adequate fluid intake assists in temporary detoxification and the temporary exclusion of food allergens. During a temporary "water fast", the administration of a well-formulated nutritional product that contains key nutrients for skin health is very valuable (Table 12). Building digestive function with prebiosis, probiosis (friendly bacteria), enzymes and detoxification (section 6) can be particularly valuable in the maintenance of cutaneous (skin and coat) health.

Many common skin disorders respond to changes in diet, especially the inclusion of raw foods. Dr. Dean Bader DVM has stressed the importance of raw food diets in healthy digestion and coat health. Our proposed formulation for skin and coat health meets the supplemental requirement for specific nutrients for skin and coat health in an ideal manner (Table 12). The formula contains digestive enzymes and probiotics (friendly bacteria) as part of its basic formulation (Table 12).

Nutritional component	Comment
Omega 3 fatty acids	Essential fatty acids are the single most important factors in skin hydration. Omega 6 fatty acids are abundant in the diet but they need to be balanced by adequate intake of omega 3 fatty acids.
Collagen	Collagen is a complex protein which contains amino acids (hydroxyproline) that are essential for building healthy connective tissue in skin. Foreign collagen can have beneficial effects on connective tissues and joints by a process of oral tolerization.

CONTINUED

Vitamins A, C and E	These classic antioxidant vitamins help protect the skin from free radical damage and each plays a special role in skin function and structure.
Vitamin B complex	The most delicious and varied natural source of many minerals and vitamins, especially vitamin B complex, is brewers yeast. Beta glucan stimulates immunity.
Probiotics/Enzymes	The maintenance of friendly bacteria in the gut (probiotics e.g. Lactobacillus) with digestive enzymes promotes skin health. Digestive function and skin health go hand in hand.
Miscellaneous:	Selenium is an antioxidant that is often deficient. Flax and wheat germ powders provide holistic vital nutrient support with balances omega 3 and 6 fatty acid precursors. Horsetail is an abundant source of silica for hair and skin health.

Table 12

The constituents of neutraceutical for skin and coat health. This formula provides an optimal array of vital nutrients for skin and coat health - see text.

General care for skin and coat health

While a good range of nutrient supplements are the mainstay of vibrant skin and coat health, several issues in general pet care are important (Table 13).

General Consideration	Comment
Skin allergies	Several topical products, especially shampoos can trigger allergies. Simple soaps are advised with the avoidance of synthetic ingredients. Allergic reactions to fleas is a common problem and severe lesions can occur around ears as a result of infestations (see Natural Ear Comfort™). Drug therapies commonly cause skin problems. Look for ringworm.
Hands on therapy	Regular grooming, cleanlines and "affection" are beneficial for skin and coat health. Avoid frequent shampooing. Brushing with a natural hair brush or dry "loofa" is a good way of stimulating skin.
Shedding	Shedding occurs as a natural cycle in animals. Removal of shed hair by grooming is very important.
Co-existing illness	Almost any disease or toxic insult to a pet can affect skin health - refer to a veterinarian to get a proper diagnosis.

Table 13
General issues in skin and coat health. Optimal nutrition is germane for skin and coat health.

The scientific basis of skin and coat formulation

Many pets with disorders of their skin and coat have allergies, especially food allergies. Food allergies can cause or contribute to poor digestive function. Veterinary scientists have recognized the importance of friendly bacteria (Probiotics) in the promotion of health in many body systems (see section 6, Digestive Health). Examples of healthy bacteria include species of the bacteria known as Lactobacillus and Bifidobacteria, especially Lactobacillus acidophilus. These friendly organisms can be given in supplements that are called probiotics (pro=for, biotics=life). Probiotic supplements have become very popular in promoting many different aspects of health (see section 6, Digestive Health).

Maintaining healthy contents of the gastrointestinal tract involves a complete diet, balancing the microflora of the bowel (friendly bacteria probiotics) and the supply of adequate amounts of digestive enzymes. Enzymes in the digestive tract are absolutely necessary for the normal absorption of nutrients. The act of supplementing the diet of pets with enzymes has been recognized as an important component in health promotion. A good skin and coat supplement contains pancreatic enzymes, which are responsible for the optimal assimilation of bodybuilding protein in the diet. The importance of probiotic and enzyme therapy in health is discussed in detail in the book entitled: "Natural Ways to Digestive Health" (Holt S., M. Evans Inc. Publishers, NY, NY, 2000).

When a primary nutritional approach to promote skin and coat health is required, antioxidant supplementation is of pivotal significance. Much research shows that environmental insults and the consequences of many diseases results in the generation of active species of chemicals in the body called "free radicals". Antioxidants, such as vitamins C or E, and essential elements, such as selenium, "mop-up" free radicals by their antioxidant effects. Vitamin A is an important fat-soluble vitamin that is required for skin health. Deficiencies of this vitamin cause skin rashes and poor function of skin cells. However, Vitamin A in high doses can be toxic and it is more suitable to take the precursor of this vitamin in the form of the antioxidant beta-carotene (Table 13).

Essential Fats

The role of essential fatty acids in general well-being is being described as an important "health link". As the name suggests, these fatty acids are "essential" and they cannot be manufactured in the body. They must come from the diet and they are as "essential" as any vitamin for health. The two types of fatty acids that are most frequently discussed are the omega 6 and omega 3 types of fatty acids. Omega 6 types are widespread in many pets' diets, but a general deficiency of omega 3 fatty acids is common (in both pets and humans). The essential fatty acids have very important roles in the support of many body functions (Table 14).

\# The normal function of the immune system.
\# Formation of substrates for hormone production and effector properties.
\# Regulation of blood pressure by involvement in vascular tone and collateral circulations.
\# Regulation of responses to pain, inflammation, infection, and cancer. Control of glandular secretion and their composition.
\# Regulation of smooth muscle and neural function.
\# Cell membrane structure and mitosis of cells.
\# Regulation of cell oxygenation and nutrient intake, the provision of energy substrates for key organs and antioxidant effects

Table 14
Effects of essential fatty acids and prostaglandins on body function.

One important issue that has emerged in nutritional medicine is the recognition of the importance of taking an adequate balance of omega 3 and 6 types of fatty acids. In and ideal supplement formulae for skin and coat health, an abundance of active omega 3 fatty acids exists in the form of stabilized fish oil (Table 14 and 15). Stabilized fish oil provides essential fatty acids of the omega 3 type that are readily utilized by the body. (See Table 16.)

The most important types of active omega 3 fatty acids are eicosapentanoic (EPA) and docosahexanoic (DHA) acids. These active types of omega 3 fatty acids help to regulate immunity, contribute to cell membrane function and they have antioxidant potential (Table 16). It is necessary to increase certain nutritional co-factors in the diet when essential fatty acids are given. In this case, an adequate supply of vitamins E, C and B complex are required. In the best supplement formula, these co-factors are supplied in a balanced way so that the health giving benefits of the essential fatty acids can be adequately realized and problems that occur with deficiency are avoided (Table 15).

The reader is cautioned that these problems are not specific to fatty acid deficiency and may occur due to other reasons (Table 15).

\#   Chronic fatigue - all symptoms encountered in chronic fatigue syndrome.

\#   Mental changes - depression, poor motivation, poor higher central nervous system function, and, perhaps, dementia.

\#   Reduced function of the immune system.

\#   Cancer and neurological disease.

\#   Cardiovascular disease, angina, high blood pressure, poor exercise tolerance.

\#   Frequent infections; e.g. colds and flu.

\#   Bone and joint problems; e.g. arthritis.

\#   Gastrointestinal upset - flatulence, constipation, and bloating.

\#   Dry skin, dry hair, cracked nails, and dry mucous membranes, e.g. eyes, mouth, and vagina.

Table 15
Signs, symptoms, and disorders attributed to essential fatty acid deficiency (LA and LNA variably).

The inclusion of wheat germ and flax seed powder in skin and coat formulae is to provide further balance of essential fatty acid precursors, which alone are not reliable sources of "active" fatty acids. Products that use flax seed as a primary source of omega 3 fatty acids are best avoided because only precursors of the acids (alpha linolenic acid) are present. Many animals are not able to convert much more than up to 10% of these precursors into the active omega 3 fatty acids, DHA and EPA.

Horsetail is a herb used for skin and coat health, because of its content of silica (Table 13). Several studies have drawn attention to the beneficial effects of silica administration on skin and hair health. The trace element selenium, is a highly versatile antioxidant, which has specific beneficial actions on protein functions in body chemistry. Selenium is a common deficiency in the diet of many animals, especially those that are maintained on commercial, cooked pet foods.

Summary

Many factors can cause poor skin and coat health. The baseline strategy for improving skin and coat health is good nutrition (Table 16). The proposed nutraceutical approach for skin and coat health has been formulated to take account of current knowledge of vital nutrients that are germane to vibrant appearances of a healthy pet (Table 16). Skin care requires a comprehensive nutraceutical, food supplement that supports skin and coat health.

Ingredient	Amount
Powdered Omega 3 fatty acids 50%	0.7 g
Collagen	275 mg
Flaxseed powder	20 mg
Wheat germ powder	20 mg
Beta Carotene	500 IU
Vitamin C	0.5 g
Vitamin E	30 mg
Horsetail	0.1 g
Selenium	2 mcg
Digestive Enzymes (pancreatin 4x)	25 mg
Lactobacillus acidophilus (5 billion CFU)	25 mg
Brewers Yeast	230.9 mg

Table 16

The above formula is a holistic mixture of essential nutrients that are valuable in the promotion of healthy skin, coat and nails or hoofs. It has an important component of silica in horsetail and it is delicious tasting for animals because of its generous content of high quality Brewers yeast, which provides essential vitamins and minerals. It has the added benefit of probiotics (Lactobacillus) and digestive enzymes. Many holistic veterinarians have indicated the importance of balanced digestive function for optimal skin and coat health. (Reproduced from www.naturesbenefit.com)

SECTION 4

Oral Health

"Take a whack at the plaque"

"Dog's breath" and "cat's breath" can be a major problem for pet owners. Much of the time, this halitosis comes from problems within the mouth, including retained food, and plaque. On occasion bad breath can signal the presence of serious oral disease or general ill health. The most common cause of persistent bad breath is sub-optimal oral hygiene. Food can get trapped between teeth and in combination with bacteria in the mouth, plaque forms and retained food "ferments". Fermented food attracts bacteria and forms a nidus for infections around teeth. The presence of tooth and adjacent gum disease (gingivitis) makes the whole process of poor oral hygiene a self-perpetuating circumstance.

When mucus, bacteria and retained food mix, plaque will form. This is a cheesy and sticky deposition around teeth and the gum margin. As this sticky plaque builds up, it hardens and forms a concretion called "tartar". Tartar is hard material that attaches strongly to teeth. When plaque and tartar build up, more bacteria tend to grow and inflammation occurs in and around the gums (gingiva) causing gingivitis.

Gingivitis is a difficult problem to treat and once it becomes established, a circumstance of periodontal disease develops. In this disorder pockets and crevices within gums and around teeth develop. With continuing inflammation and infection, a "viscous cycle" of poor dental health is set up in the pet.

Periodontal disease and dangers to your pet

Given this sequence of events, it is unfortunate that many pets are left to develop severe plaque and tartar formation. Plaque and tartar has to be treated in many cases by scaling. In this situation, the pet has to be put to sleep with anesthesia, whilst the teeth are scraped with steel instruments and irrigated with a water pik. In severe situations, the veterinarian has to cut out pieces of infected gums, in order that healing can occur.

Many cats develop serious gingivitis, which is sometimes so severe that it is treated with corticosteroids to reduce inflammation. The use of steroids in this circumstance is questionable. Persian and Himalayan cats seem particularly susceptible to this severe form of gingivitis, which sometimes interferes with eating. Steroids often do not work in this situation and they weaken immune function. Antibiotics work variably, but they will disturb the friendly bacteria of the gut and they have other undesirable side effects.

Component	Comment
Soluble fiber	When soluble fiber comes into contact with water it forms a sticky gel that will stick to teeth and the gum margins on a temporary basis.
Enzymes	Mixed proteolytic enzymes, papain from papaya tends to break down protein strands, loosening sticky plaque.
Vitmain C and Green Tea extract	These natural substances are powerful antioxidants.
Grain alcohol	Grain alcohol is a preservative and an antiseptic.

Table 17
Components of an oral biocleansing system

This terrible situation of poor oral health puts the pet at risk of anesthesia for scaling. Surgery performed on an infected mouth can cause transition of infection (spread) elsewhere in the body.

Clearly, the solution is to avoid this situation. There are several natural ways to oral health that have been proposed and many are ideally focused on plaque prevention. The simplest, novel, convenient and cost effective way to deal with this situation is the use of oral biocleansing with enzymes and antioxidants (Table 17). This forms the basis of a unique, oral biocleansing system.

Further understanding oral hygiene

Poor oral hygiene and/or the common occurrence of gum or gingival disease (gingivitis) are the main causes of bad breath in pets. Gingivitis is often classified under the term "periodontal disease". Airflows freely through the mouth, nasal passages, throat area, and respiratory passages of the lungs. Diseases that involve inflammation or tissue damage at any site along the passage of air into the body can cause a foul odor, but the mouth is usually the origin of bad breath in animals. In cases of doubt about the source of halitosis, a veterinary consultation is required.

To briefly review the circumstances, inflammation and disorders of the gums and teeth that result in gingivitis and gum pockets are classic examples of periodontal disease. When periodontal disease becomes established, the gums drift away from their junction with the teeth. Mixed infections occur around the lower areas of the teeth at their junction with the gums and this disorder is often associated with the presence of dental plaque. Plaque is a "cheesy" concretion that becomes deposited between and around the teeth. Left alone, plaque sets like liquid concrete and results in tartar. Plaque prevention and removal is a pivotal step in maintaining oral health.

To reiterate, pockets often form around gums and bacteria, food fragments and plaque can collect in these pockets or grooves. Sometimes the gums can swell and bleed. Enlargement of the gums may be quite pronounced and surgical correction is required sometimes by a periodontist (a dental surgeon who specializes in these problems). However, it is often possible to avoid the dental surgeon's scalpel by practicing periodontal hygiene. The mainstay of conventional management of periodontal disease involves plaque removal by brushing, flossing, and the scaling techniques used by a dental hygienist. Brushing cats 'or dogs' teeth is not fun for anyone!

Teeth are perched in alveolar bones and anchored by ligaments. A tooth has an enamel coating covering soft tissue called dentin. Damage to enamel causes cavities in the teeth. Many factors play a role in preventing tooth decay. Saliva is very important in maintaining healthy teeth and gums. It is alkaline and buffers excess acid, serving the purpose of irrigation of the mouth, fighting infections and maintaining the proper degree of mineral content of teeth.

One of the most destructive influences on teeth is the presence of acidity in the mouth. The pH of the mouth falls (acidity) as a result of the action of bacteria on food particles that are retained along the dental margin. This explains why drinks of low pH (soda) are damaging. Excessive sugar is bad for teeth - bacteria love sugar and so do our pets! Bacteria and food particles work together to cause plaque, which can collect as soon as four to six hours, even after brushing the teeth. If left, plaque attracts mineral and bacteria to form tartar, a form of hard material (yellowish, dental concrete) that sticks to the teeth. The build up of plaque and tartar is related to the types of plaque-forming bacteria present in the mouth and rates of flow of saliva. The characteristics of the pet's diet play a major role in maintaining oral health. Remember, sugar is a real miscreant, watch those candies!

More about bad breath

The throat area (pharynx) is a shared route to both the lungs and the upper gastrointestinal tract. In this region, upper gastrointestinal air is exposed to exhaled breath. Any strong-smelling food that has been eaten recently can be readily detected on the breath. Spices and fish are common causes of breath odor following meals. If food hangs around in the stomach or upper gastrointestinal tract, it can ferment or putrefy. Food that hangs around in the guts attracts unwanted guests in the form of harmful bacteria and microorganisms. Probiotic and enzyme therapy can help in this situation (see section 6), but biocleansing the mouth is very important.

As well as the common occurrence of odors from pungent foods, other gases or volatile compounds can be present in the breath. Volatile fatty acids can emanate from the guts in states of disease. Liver failure or kidney failure can give rise to chemicals that are part of body waste. These include ammonia-based compounds that can result in halitosis. Odors in the breath can come from sites distant from the respiratory or digestive passages. A number of aromatic substances when applied to the body can be detected in the breath. Experiments performed sixty years ago showed that when garlic was rubbed on the soles of the feet, its odor appeared in the breath!

One big problem in some pets is licking areas of the body such as "private parts". These areas carry odors that may linger in the pet's breath. Excessive licking of body parts may signal local injury or a behavioral problem in animals. It can be caused by stress or separation anxiety (see Section 5, Behavioral Problems). During normal grooming, cats and dogs can transfer odors from their coat to their mouth. Some of this behavior is normal pet behavior and attempts to extinguish it should not be made. Extinguishing normal behavior in animals leads to complex behavioral problems.

Breath fresheners

Freshening the breath of pets is big business. A whole host of products are purveyed to assure fresh breath in pets, but few work. One has a choice of flavored "candies", sprays, tablets, lozengers, mouth rinses, and drinks. Pets find this approach to odor control unpleasant and substances like peppermint can cause cats and dogs to foam at the mouth (hyper salivation). The problem is that most of these "breath fresheners" are quite ineffective, or, at best, they will substitute a strong pleasant odor for a bad odor, only for a matter of a few minutes. Sometimes an attempt to disguise bad breath with a volatile oil or flavor used in these products can result in a combined odor that is worse than the original odor!

Internal deodorization

We all want to be assured that our pet smells good. In states of health, the pet's body can disguise its own natural odors, but it always needs a bit of help. According to popular advertising, help comes in the form of the perfumes, deodorants, and cosmetics. But the superficial odor from these products will not disguise the smell of poor oral or general health of a pet. Many pet perfumes or cosmetics contain synthetic additives that can be damaging to your pet - please read labels. There are several valuable natural pet deodorizers of freshening sprays for the home. The highest quality is made by "Pet-Air", California.

The knowledge that gastrointestinal disturbance can cause bad breath has prompted people to think of the concept of internal deodorization, and many natural techniques have been applied. I believe that odors from the guts are often due to an imbalance of the inhabitants of the guts, where friendly bacteria are ousted or substituted by unwanted guests. Probiotic therapy (treatment using friendly bacteria) has a lot to offer in counteracting unpleasant gut odors (see section 6 and section 3).

Swollen, bleeding gums

Swollen and bleeding gums are "red flag signs" in many circumstances. This condition in a pet must be taken seriously. While it is often due to gingivitis, it can be the first sign of serious disease, such as cancers of the blood or immunodeficiencies. Swollen and bleeding gums should prompt and individual to seek consultation with a veterinarian.

Diseases and oral health

Thirty years ago, Professor Samuel C. Miller, D.D.S., of the New York School of Dentistry proposed a relationship between poor dental hygiene and many different diseases in animals and humans. His work was ignored for a decade, until these relationships were further examined. In particular, there seems to be a close link between a variety of chronic diseases and dental health, e.g. cardiovascular, digestive and joint disease.

Several studies reported in the medical literature indicate the possibility of bacterial translocation from the mouth (migration and travel of bacteria) to bloodstream. This forms part of the well-recognized disease links between the mouth and the rest of the body. Bacteria that are found in the mouth can collect in atheromatous plaques (cholesterol deposits) that are found in arteries throughout the body, especially in humans. Organisms that have been identified as being able to travel from the mouth to the body include Helicobacter pylori (associated with gastritis and peptic ulcer) and Chlamydia pneumoniae (a common cause of lung infection).

In animal experiments performed at the University of Minnesota, dental research showed that bacteria from dental plaque were able to escape into the bloodstream and produce small blood clots in animals. In these experiments, large amounts of certain bacteria (Streptococcus sanguis and Porphyromonas gingivalis - common oral inhabitants) caused irregular heartbeats and early signs of a heart attack. It appears that these common mouth bacteria have clotting factors on their surface that cause blood to coagulate (especially common with Streptococcus sanguis).

Studies at the University of Toronto, Canada, have shown the presence of immune markers that are derived from oral bacteria in cholesterol-containing plaques in arterial blood vessels (atherosclerosis). This indicates a potential relationship between oral bacteria and arteriosclerosis (hardening of the arteries). These findings are supported by human, population studies that links the presence of gum disease with the occurrence of cardiovascular disease, coronary heart disease, and stroke in humans and animals.

The associations of poor dental hygiene and heart disease have been extended to lung disease, impaired immunity and peptic ulcer disease. Overall, it seems that dental health is much a more important regulator of general health than medicine has previously recognized. Poor oral health plays a major role in the cause of several, severe diseases. Keeping the mouth clean breaks the "oral - body" disease link.

Natural enzymatic digest and biocleansing

Prevention of oral disease must concentrate on a variety of issues affecting oral health, including: oral hygiene, the nature of plaque forming bacteria, retained food residue in the mouth, salivary flora (bacteria or yeasts), general immunity, and nutritional or dietary habits. The sequence in which some foods are eaten and the interval between their consumption has been shown to be important. For instance, if bone meal is eaten shortly after a sugary item, the acid formed from the sugar is neutralized by the bone meal.

Oral hygiene in humans and many pets involves meticulous attention to the gums, teeth and mouth. Some methods of oral hygiene are expensive, time consuming, and often poorly undertaken. In order to simplify the approach to oral cleanliness, a rapid and effective way of cleaning the mouth with an enzymatic digest gel has been developed in the form of an oral biocleansing system (Table 15). This system is not toothpaste, it is a gel that is based on completely natural ingredients.

This novel enzymatic gel has a base of soluble fiber that "holds water" and is quite sticky. Its sticky nature is desirable so that it is well attached to the teeth and gum margin where it exerts its cleansing effects. Added to the base of "sticky fiber" are enzymes from fruit (papain, from papaya). When this natural enzyme is contained in a matrix of sticky fiber and rubbed on the teeth, it loosens and partially dissolves plaque and debris around the teeth. In order to enhance the mouth "cleanup" and control of bacteria, several natural agents are added that have powerful antioxidant actions. These natural additives include green tea extract and vitamin C (Table 15).

The use of vitamin C for dental health has been undervalued. In one study, vitamin C supplementation of the diet in young boys resulted in a cleaner mouth, regardless of how well or how poorly these boys brushed their teeth! It appears that vitamin C is quite important in the prevention of gingivitis. Vitamin C exerts its beneficial effects on oral hygiene by its antioxidant effects. Effective oral cleansing systems also contain green tea extract. The value of green tea as a powerful antioxidant is well recognized and it is inhibitory against the growth of certain bacteria and the damage they can cause to tissue by oxidative stress (free radical generation). Green tea extracts are used widely in Eastern Asia, especially Japan, as ways of promoting good oral hygiene.

Summary

Oral health in animals is a very common problem that can place a pet at great risk of serious disease. Preventing gingivitis, excessive plaque and tartar formation is a key issue in health maintenance in pets. Poor oral hygiene often results in bad breath in dogs and cats. Keeping teeth clean by brushing etc. is difficult in many pets. Alternative ways of ensuring mouth hygiene and reduction of plaque formation by oral biocleansing is a very attractive option. Oral biocleansing is easier to use than standard enzymatic toothpastes and it sticks to teeth to extend its duration of cleansing action. The revolutionary, enzymatic, antioxidant-cleansing system used in oral biocleansers may greatly contribute to oral health and reduction in the "oral disease – body disease link". It can help to avoid unpleasant breath odors from a pet's mouth that may make "closeness" with your loved companion sometimes undesirable.

Behavioral Problems

Pets have emotions and "feelings"

If humans cannot recognize the feelings and emotions of their own pet, they should join the other members of the flat earth society! Some veterinarians can be slim on advice about behavioral problems in animals and the guidance of experienced trainers or pet owners is often very valuable. The limited studies that exist on behavioral problems in dogs indicate that causes include: lack of knowledge about the pet's basic needs or nature, poor or absent training routines and a lack of structure in day-to-day activity. One important cause of behavioral problems in cats or dogs or horses is the owner's behavior! We do not wish to sound harsh, but we all have a responsibility to understand the social and psychological needs of our pets.

Medical disorders that causes poor behavior

Not all problems with pet's behavior are caused by social or environmental issues. Almost any disease that distresses a pet may result in change of behavior. It is often advisable in cases of an abrupt change in the personality of a pet to seek consultation with a veterinarian. Disorders such as mite or flea infestations, ear problems, urinary tract infections or serious disease can be at the root of adverse actions or behavior displayed by your pet.

Some common causes of behavior change result from the normal physiology of a pet. Change in normal hormone cycles, such as excessive testosterone surges in males and "going into heat" in females, often alter a dog's or cat's temperament. With advances in environmental medicine, veterinarians have learned a great deal about the role of "household toxins" in changing a pet's behavior. These toxins range from cleaning fluids to the artificial additives found in some pet foods.

Pets with anxiety, pain or discomfort can engage sometimes in very bizarre behavior. They may forget their domestic training and soil. Some will chase their tail repeatedly or shake their head in a dangerous way (see section 8, Ear Health). A "funny" kind of behavior is scooting, where a dog rubs its rear end along the floor. This may be a sign of local irritation to tail end (anal area) and it is often caused by problems with anal glands. However, scooting can arise from discomfort elsewhere in the body e.g. ear or skin irritations. Any sign of self-destructive behavior in a pet must be taken very seriously.

Managing poor behavior

The primary approach to correct poor behavior is a "behavioral approach". Certain strategies are important, especially in the management of separation anxiety or conditioning to events that trigger bad behavior. Advances in psychoneuronutrition (psycho=mind, neuro=nervous system) underscore the importance of correct nutrition in optimal pet behavior. A well balanced diet with extra nutrient supplements is often enough to reverse the behavior problem of a pet in some circumstances. Dogs that are not "satisfied" with their diet will behave like they are "starving". This leads to "trash rooting", chewing and disturbance of normal behavior patterns.

Certain nutrients are vital for brain and mind function. In some circumstances, nutrients can play a role in mood. For example, modern research at Harvard University and Baylor College of Medicine, in Houston, Texas, has shown that certain essential fatty acids (omega 3 types in fish oil) can act like an "antidepressant". Of particular significance are the findings of essential fatty acid deficiency in dogs and cats, especially fats of the omega 3 series. It is known that the central nervous system of all animals is composed mainly of unsaturated fats, especially docosahexanoic acid (DHA) and eicosapentanoic acid (EPA). These two types of omega 3 fat (DHA and EPA) are examples of active fatty acids that are found in their "active" format in fish oil.

There has been much written in natural medicine about omega 3 factors in the diet and popular products based on plant sources of omega 3 fatty acids (e.g. flax seed) have been used increasingly. It is very important to realize that plant sources of omega 3 fatty acids contain only precursors of EPA and DHA and many dogs or cats may not be able to adequately convert these precursors in flax into the active types of fatty acids. Therefore, the most effective sources of active omega 3 fatty are fish oil, which are readily available in some products in a dry, stabilized, powder format (see section 7). Omega 3 fatty acids from fish oil are useful in skin formulae (section 3) and the support of healthy immune function (section 7).

The value of omega 3 fatty acids in supporting brain structure and function is well described in the scientific literature. Favorable observations on omega 3 supplementation with fish oil for behavioral problems in dogs are consistent with similar observations on the beneficial effects of omega 3 fatty acid supplementation on attention deficit disorder in children and adults. Balanced sources of the omega factors must be sought and they are readily available in dietary supplement format (see The Immune Factor, section 7).

Ancillary support for bad behavior

Adequate exposure of a dog to unfiltered, natural light and regular exercise are absolutely necessary for good health and behavior. Animals respond to the joy of play and companionship. Dogs are pack animals and they like dens. The creation of a "little house" or secure area for your dog in a basket or "penned area" is often quite comforting. Cats like little "hiding places" where they can exercise their traits of independence, in privacy. Some individuals think that a dog should not have a restrained environment, but their instincts are for intermittent privacy and security.

A number of alternative management approaches to a behavior include homeopathic remedies, hydrotherapy and "hands on" treatments such as touch therapy, acupuncture and massage. Whilst these approaches are often valuable, the response is variable. A consistent response in cases of stress, anxiety and "bad behavior" can often be achieved by the use of well-formulated herbal and botanical food supplements. Certain remedies of natural origin can help allay anxiety and create mood changes whilst behavior modification techniques are applied over a period of time (Table 18).

Whilst a loving and secure environment with consistent discipline can result in optimal behavior of pets, there are many circumstances that aggravate or precipitate undesirable behavioral traits. Under these circumstances, veterinarians in conventional practice have used sedatives, tranquilizers and mood altering drugs. Whilst such drugs act efficiently, they possess many disadvantages or limitations including "hangover" effects and other significant adverse side effects. Sedatives can on occasion dull senses of a pet to a level where signals from its environment are distorted and stress may actually increase. Rather than help to correct poor behavior in this situation, the drugs may tend promote the occurrence of bad behavior.

Vital Nutrients

Vitamin B complex and trace micronutrients found in Brewer's yeast. Magnesium is a "relaxing" element. Good protein sources.

Valerian, Chamomile, Kava, St. Johns Wort, Ashwaganda, Passion Flower, Lemon balm, Catnip (dual excitement or tranquility), Scullcap

Table 18

A group of vital nutrients and plant substances that have a well described role in influencing animal and human behavior. These agents have all been used in veterinary, holistic health practice.

Behavioral approaches

There are many great books written on behavior modification in pets. Pets are often much more intelligent than we suppose. They are eager to learn and their learning is always reinforced by kindness. If your pet behaves well make sure you reward the behavior by affection and an occasional "treat" (but watch those teeth!). Not all animals are compliant, some are very proud, cats are often "independent" and on occasion your pet can be just as stubborn as you, especially when they are anxious or disturbed. Learning to communicate with your pet is very important. Animals have complex patterns of non-verbal communication. Look closely at their posture, eye movements and facial expressions. A lot can be learned by careful watching.

A very common and underestimated problem for our loved companions is separation anxiety. Anxiety or stress is caused in this situation by the loss of the owner's presence. In some respects, it can be seen as a state of deprivation. We can learn a great deal from the study of separation anxiety in humans. During childhood development, separation anxiety is most pronounced in children between the age of one and two years. Even brief separation of a mother from a baby can cause great anxiety for a child. We want pet owners to understand this circumstance in their own pet. The owner is the center of attention for the pet and the loyal pet will always react to their owner's absence to a variable degree. This is a sign of the love your pet has for you and the power of your bond with your companion animal.

Separation Anxiety is common

It is estimated that seven million dogs, and perhaps as many cats, suffer from separation anxiety. "Horse jitters" are often soothed by the presence of their owner. Sometimes the condition of separation anxiety is hard to spot or it confuses a pet owner into believing that their pet may be sick with a physical illness. Obvious signs or symptoms of separation anxiety can involve: barking, whining (excessive "meows" in cats), destroying the environment, "tics", self destructive acts, head banging and indiscriminate wetting or pooping etc. Unfortunately, this kind of behavior can distress owners to a point that may even part with their pet. We must avoid this circumstance, because too many pets end up in adoption programs, which lead to their death, if a new owner does not come along. Please work with your pet to avoid parting.

So serious is separation anxiety that several drug therapies have been proposed for its treatment. Again, many pet owners prefer simple, safer, gentler, natural alternatives to drugs and their unfortunate side effects (Table 18). Medical authors have written a great deal about behavior modification in humans as part of lifestyle adjustments for health (see Holt S., The Natural Way to a Healthy Heart, Evans and Co. Publishers, NY, NY, 1999). Just like in humans, antecedent (preceding) cues precipitate bad behavior in pets, which should not be rewarded. A principal cue for bad behavior in pets is an owner's absence.

We shall examine the possibility of using nutrients and botanical agents as part of natural interventions for poor behavior, but behavioral training programs must be instituted with your companion. It is important to remove obvious stressors from your pet's environment. When you leave home, the placement of your pet in the correct location in the home is very important. If animals are too confined they are stressed and, in turn, if left to roam they are provoked or encounter stressful situations.

Simple advice on leaving your pet

Some simple advice for leaving dogs and cats at home can be followed. It is important not to focus attention on your pet for about 15-30 minutes prior to you leaving the home. The pet owner's departure should be "low key". Just leave with an air of "matter of fact". Fond farewells for animals can reinforce separation anxiety. It is useful to make a "toy" a focus of your departure. The "toy" is a signal to your pet that you are leaving, but it is reassuring if you take the toy away when you come home. The toy becomes a token of comfort. This kind of routine can be highly effective in allaying anxiety.

One significant issue is to ignore your pet, if it greets you with excessive excitement. Patting and praising a jumping dog or naughty cat just reinforces the behavior you want to go away. Acknowledge your pet when they have settled down. It is very important not to punish bad behavior "after the fact". Signs of disapproval must be expressed to a pet at the time of the occurrence of the bad behavior. If you follow these guidelines, problems will be lessened, but sometimes your pet will need help and this can be achieved in a natural way (Table 18). Remember herbs are best used with advice from a veterinarian.

The natural approach to stress and anxiety control

A variety of natural herbals and botanicals have been proposed as valuable in the correction of stress, anxiety and disturbed behavior in animals (Table 18). Each natural agent mentioned in Table 18 has a long history of use in "nurturing" the brain, natural tranquilizing and suppression of anxiousness. The nutrient content of food supplements to relax pets (cats and dogs) includes the B complex vitamins and trace elements found in Brewer's yeast. Added to the holistic formulae is the calming effect of magnesium, which facilitates the normal functions of muscle relaxation. To promote proper neurotransmitter function (molecules of communication), vitamins of the B complex are valuable (present in Brewer's yeast).

The presence of desiccated liver or other foods in formulae can provide other vital nutrients, including vitamin B12.

Much has been written about the psychoactive effects (mind effects) of many herbals. Those herbs or botanicals with well-described effects on mood and behavior are present in many mixes. They include valerian, chamomile, Kava kava, St. John's Wort, Ashwaganda, Passion flower, Lemon balm, Catnip and Scullcap. Each of these plant fractions has very specific and valuable effects on mood and behavior. These components are found in supplements used as nutritional support to relax pets and their special properties require a brief review (Table 18).

Valerian (Valeriana officinalis)

Valerian root is a pungent herb with an unpleasant smell that actually attracts dogs. Herbalists have used valerian extensively as a minor sedative and it is useful for states of excitation, nervous anxiety and insomnia. It assists the body in general relaxation and it is quite valuable as a sedative in the presence of stress, discomfort or pain.

On a practical basis, valerian is very useful for minor sedation, when a pet is traveling or when environmental stress is present e.g. fireworks, heavy traffic noises, strange surroundings, during grooming and after surgical procedures. In addition to this sedative action, valerian root has anticonvulsant activity. It depresses the nervous system in a gentle manner at moderate doses and it may prevent seizures.

Careful scientific studies show that valerian interferes with the function of certain molecules that pass messages in the brain and nervous system. It inhibits the enzymatic breakdown of the neurotransmitter gamma-amino-butyric acid, GABA. Valerian is suitable for repeated administration over several days and many pet owners have found it useful to give valerian in modest doses for a week or two before a stressful event such as extended kennel care (when owners are on vacation) or when a major trip or event is planned.

Valerian has been used safely in cats, dogs and horses, but large amounts of valerian may cause vomiting and it is best avoided during pregnancy. Valerian seems to have useful properties for relaxing smooth muscle in the bowel and it helps in cats and dogs who have irritability of their digestive tracts. Some pets respond to the stresses or pressures of life with digestive upsets e.g. soiling during separation anxiety.

Chamomile (Matricara recutita)

Chamomile has been widely used as a mild sedative, and it has smooth muscle relaxing activity. Smooth muscle is found in the organs of the digestive tract. It is particularly valuable for digestive upset that occurs with nervousness, stress and excitement. Chamomile is a complex mixture of bioactive compounds, many of which function as "antispasmodics" (relieve colic or spasm in the gut). It is a tried and trusted remedy for anxiety and its related behavioral associations. This general purpose and versatile herb is ideal for inclusion in herbal formulae to assist in managing difficult behavioral problems.

Kava Kava

Kava Kava is a very interesting psychoactive herb that originates in specific locations in the temperate Pacific islands. Much Kava is grown and used in the South Pacific islands e.g. Kuauai. This herb has become very popular as a safe anxiolytic and it has been likened to a safe, natural form of tranquilizer. Kava is well tolerated in modest doses but in high doses, with long-term use, it can cause an unusual skin rash, which has been described rarely in humans.

Kava (Piper methysticum) is now popular in Western society as a mild sedative and reducer of feelings of anxiety. The active components of Kava are believed to be the Kavalactones. Well-controlled, clinical trials have shown that Kava can control symptoms of anxiety, enhance memory, improve reaction time and lead to greater vigilance. It is the whole root complex that seems to be a holistic, mild sedative that does not cause drowsiness.

St. John's Wort

St. John's Wort has been called nature's blues-buster because of its well-defined antidepressant effects. The active components of St. John's Wort are compounds called hyperforins and hypericins. Clinical studies in humans imply that St. John's Wort may be as valuable as many anti-depressant drugs and it has been used widely for its calming and mood elevating properties in humans.

St. John's Wort is a widely researched, natural antidepressant.

In fact, more than 1500 human patients have been studied in greater than twenty controlled clinical trials with evidence of overall benefit. It has few side effects, the most common of which is minor digestive upset. Some studies comparing the use of St. John's Wort with antidepressant drugs show comparable benefits in elevation of mood, but in the case of St. John's Wort, side effects were minimal. Spotting depression in pets is difficult but you should have no doubt that it occurs.

Ashwaganda (Withania somnifera)

Ashwaganda is an herb with a long-standing use in Ayurvedic medicine, where it is used as a general "nerve" tonic. The discipline of Ayurvedic medicine is one of the most ancient forms of traditional medicine, developed more than a couple of thousand years ago. It is very interesting to note the word Ashwagandha means "vitality of the horse" in ancient Sanskrit language. The root of the plant is used and it is sometimes called "winter cherry". The plant grows at elevated positions of about 6000 feet, especially in the Himalayan Mountains.

Ashwagandha has been used most often as an "adaptogenic" herb (balancing) with general tonic actions. It is believed to be particularly valuable in elderly humans and animals when general debility is present. Its general benefits are best understood by the reference to ashwagandha as the example of "Indian Ginseng".

There have been many studies of the use of ashwagandha root in Ayurvedic healing and it is becoming increasingly popular in North America. To summarize its actions, ashwagandha is referred to in Ayurvedic medicine as: a nervine (cf scullcap), an astringent, a rejuvenating herb, a sedative, a tonic and an aphrodisiac. It is an herb that helps to build several body functions in states of nervous debility whilst allaying anxiety by its mild sedative actions.

Passion Flower

Passionflower extracts have enjoyed most use as a minor tranquilizer and they have been used extensively in folklore medicine as a female tonic. Preparations of passionflower are made from the flowers, leaves and fruit of the creeping vine (Passiflora incarnata). The real use of passionflower is as an adaptogen or a substance that helps "balance" the body, especially in terms of the function of the nervous system. Passionflower can be used in females to calm the mind that may be disturbed by periods of repeated hormonal adjustments that occur in women. Thus, passionflower is particularly useful in calming a female animal who is "in heat" (estrous). Although passionflower has been recognized as being of particular value in females, it exerts useful calming effects in males.

Passionflower is regarded as an effective remedy for nerves that are on edge. J. Lutomski, M.D., has drawn attention to the balance brought to females by passionflower in his paper. *Die Bedeutung der Passionsblume in der Heilkunde,* published in the journal. Pharmazie in unserer Zeit, in 1981. (10,2, pp.45-49). Roughly translated, the title of this paper is *"The Meaning of Passion Flower in Current Times."* The tranquilizing benefits of passionflower are particularly useful in nervous manifestations of menstrual problems, and menopause in humans and animals. There are no known side effects or contraindications to passionflower, according to Dr. Varro Tyler in his famous book *"Herbs of Choice."*

Lemon balm (Melissa officinalis)

Lemon balm is derived from a plant that grows mainly in the Eastern Mediterranean and the Western parts of Asia. It contains a number of essential oils and polyphenolic compounds. Its effects are wide-ranging and very interesting. The herb in its common form of lemon balm is a sedative with antispasmodic actions. In naturopathic medicine, it is highly regarded as an antibacterial agent. It has been employed most often for gastrointestinal and cardiovascular disorders that are nervous in origin. It is a classic "nervine". Experiments in mice have shown lemon balm to have both sedative and painkilling effects.

Extensive accounts of its use in folklore medicine describe its calming ability without the occurrence of a "hangover". It has been regarded as particularly valuable in states of melancholia (sadness) and hysteria (extreme agitation). This makes lemon balm very valuable for the nervous or dependent pet. It has been noted to deal with rapid heart beat (palpitations) that are precipitated by nervousness. Whilst lemon balm is calming, it is also described as a "strenghtening" remedy. It has an interesting ability to correct nervous disorders that interfere with sleep and it can correct anxiety-induced effects on the gut. In circumstances of debility, lemon balm has been useful at stimulating appetite. The herb is regarded as quite safe and particularly valuable in circumstances of separation anxiety, "jitters" whilst traveling and excitement induced by changes in the environment of a pet.

Catnip (Nepeta cateria)

Catnip is an intriguing herb that holds special fascination for cats. Catnip acts generally as a mild tranquilizer or sedative that allays anxiety and helps promote restful sleep in many animals. It is generally believed that catnip excites cats and this is true if they sniff the herb for significant amounts of time. In fact, some cats who sniff catnip may behave as though they are "drunk" (intoxicated).

When catnip is taken as an oral herb, it does not tend to cause euphoria in the same way that occurs as a consequence of "sniffing". Catnip has a special role in settling the stomach and bowels of "nervous" animals. As mentioned, some animals respond with digestive upset (diarrhea or vomiting) to stress in their environment and in these animals, catnip can work "like a charm". Herbalists report the value of catnip as a "social herb" when animals are introduced to each other, especially if a cat is exposed to a new companion e.g. a dog or another cat.

Scullcap (Scutellaria laterifolia)

Scullcap belongs to the "mint" family of plants and it has sedative, anxiolytic and anticonvulsant properties. It is referred to by herbalists as a "nervine" because of its special actions on the nervous system. For many years, Scullcap has been used to treat acute and chronic nervous disorders where anxiety predominates.

Scullcap seems to have versatile actions on the nervous system. It calms "jittery animals", but it does not cause drowsiness. The herb has been called an "adaptogen" because of its ability to calm or balance nervous behavior in animals, without inducing sleep. During times of rehabilitation from injury, scullcap appears to have special value. It helps an animal feel calm but does not dull the senses. Scullcap is particularly valuable in separation anxiety. Scullcap is not advised in pregnancy or in the presence of significant liver disease. Note not all botanicals are always safe.

Unpredictable effects from psychoactive herbs

The description of the effects of each herb in recommended formulae is based on the usual reaction of pets to the specific herbs. However, on occasion, a strange, contrarian behavioral effect may occur in some dogs, cats or horses. For example. Valerian usually causes a sedative effect but, infrequently, it can cause an excitatory effect. Pet owners are advised to test animals' reactions to small amounts of psychoactive herbs, if they are used for the first time. In general, these herbs are quite safe, but they are best avoided in pregnancy. In cases of doubt, please check with a veterinarian.

Gadgets for "bad behavior"

There are a number of special products (gadgets) that are used in behavior training. Unfortunately, many are expensive and some are quite impractical. Indoor and outdoor animal houses (kennels) are valuable and odor control or producing products can help with housetraining. One of the most important issues is consistency of an owner's behavior and the development of pet routines. Cats love "scratching posts", but it is surprising how pet owners often fail to recognize this simple need. An old piece of rug on a fallen tree branch is ideal.

Veterinarians and trainers can give advice about the suitability of sophisticated gadgets for behavior training. The use of harnesses, head restraints and specialized techniques of behavior conditioning require expert advice from a veterinarian.

Summary

Getting along with your pet shares many features of getting along with people. Good communication, with consistent and appropriate interactions, assisted by behavior therapies and natural agents work most of the time. Love your pet and they will return the affection with greater magnitude. If doubt exists, not only love your pet, but visit your vet!

SECTION 6

Digestive Health

Natural Ways to Digestive Health

In the book, *Natural Ways to Digestive Health* (M. Evans Publishers Inc., NY, NY, 2000), Dr. Holt raises the importance of gastrointestinal function as a regulator of health in every organ in the body. The gastrointestinal tract (gut) has a careful job to do in absorbing vital nutrients, keeping out unwanted guests (antigens) and maintaining its own, well-balanced environment. In natural medicine, we have learned about the importance of supply of enzymes for digestion and the promotion of the growth of friendly bacteria in the bowel (probiosis). The process of seeding the intestines with friendly bacteria that are normally found in healthy intestines is called "probiotic therapy".

Probiosis

A century ago, Dr. Elias Metchnikoff was awarded a Nobel Prize for his work on probiosis (pro=for and biosis= life). The far-reaching health consequences of the maintenance of the right kind of bacteria in the bowel were recognized by Metchnikoff and termed "probiosis". This health giving potential of friendly bacteria is now recognized by conventional medicine. In January 2000, the American Journal of Gastroenterology produced a special monograph on "probiotics" (friendly bacteria) and their beneficial use in a variety of diseases including: immunodeficiency (HIV), inflammatory bowel disease and gut infections. What may have once been considered alternative medicine with the application of feeding friendly bacteria ("probiosis") is now "main-line" medicine.

Friendly and unfriendly inhabitants of the bowel

There are a variety of microorganisms that are characterized as friendly to the host. Some of these bacteria occupy the bowel and play a protective role against the growth of unfriendly microorganisms. Friendly bacteria in the gut can help digestive processes in general. These friendly bacteria (probiotics) have many beneficial functions including the elaboration of natural antibiotic substances that can kill other bacteria and an ability to detoxify (metabolize) toxins taken in the diet or generated in the bowel itself (Table 19). One important and underestimated action of friendly bacteria is their ability to maintain healthy immune function in the body and gut (Table 19). Friendly bacteria will help the gut to work against parasites.

The act of direct feeding of friendly bacteria is called probiotic therapy. Lactobacillus acidophilus and bulgaricus were the first bacteria to be shown to exert the symbiotic (living together with benefit) relationship that gives the body a chance to develop a healthy environment in the gut. A healthy flora in the gut can assist in both disease prevention and treatment. There have been hundreds of scientific studies in animals and humans that show the ability of Lactobacillus acidophilus to aid digestion, supply nutrients to the body, fight off infection and promote general health of many body organs (Table 19).

The friendly bacteria in our pets' bowels function to fight the unfriendly bacteria, but, we stress again that they are necessary for the maintenance of "balance" of many body functions. The widespread use of antibiotics, the occurrence of toxins in the diet and even stress, illness or injury can alter the healthy microflora of the digestive tract (bacterial environment of the gut). This situation leads to many health problems. The gut may become "leaky" and food allergies appear, immunity can be impaired and chronic disease can emerge as a consequence of removing "normal", healthy bacterial inhabitants of the bowel (the friendly bacteria, Table 19).

Benefit	Comment
Synthesize vitamins	Not all strains of Lactobacilli have this advantage. L. acidophilus synthesizes folic acid, vit. B6, B12, niacin, and riboflavin.
Enhances digestibility of foods	Lactobacilli and Bifidobacteria produce enzymes that can split food and reduce some symptoms of sad guts.
Helps lactose intolerance	Lactose is the mils sugar that is broken down by lactase. Lactase is secreted by Lactobacilli.
Suppresses gut pathogenic organisms	Natural antibiotics and resistance factors suppress unwanted bacteria and the yeast Candida albicans.
Reduces blood cholesterol	Acidophilus produces antilipidemic factors.
Functional disorders of the gut	More research required but studies are promising, e.g. halitosis, irregular bowel habit.
Traveler's diarrhea	Good trial results.
Gut infections	Strong evidence for benefit emerging.
Enhances immune function	Shown in clinical trials in humans and animals.

Table 19
Summary of some of the reported benefits of friendly bacteria (Lactobacilli and Bifidobacteria) and comments about the implications of the benefits.

In veterinary practice, many circumstances are encountered where the gut microflora becomes disturbed or unbalanced, with the loss of friendly bacteria. These situations include antibiotic treatments, parasite infestations, changes in diet, nutritional deficiencies, giving birth, body changes during weaning (problems for pups and kittens), overexertion, prolonged kennel housing and, of course, exposure to microorganisms that cause infection. Therefore, there are many circumstances for a pet when probiotic therapy becomes very valuable (Table 20).

Assistance with digestion

- Allevation of digestive disorders, e.g. colitis, IBS, peptic ulcer.
- Enhancement of the synthesis of several vitamins (especially B complex).
- Protection against pathogenic bacterial infections, e.g. E. Coli infection.
- Reduction of symptoms of lactose intolerance permits limited reintroduction of dairy products.
- Reduction of yeast overgrowth (candidiasis), notable reduction in thrush.
- Improvement in immune function, "primes" the gut immune system.
- Anticarcinogenic effects, some good evidence.
- Prevention of Helicobactor pylori infection and its association with peptic ulcer. (humans)

Table 20
Proposed major benefits of probiotic therapy.

More benefits of probiotics

The "stress" responses that we have described above that alter the flora of the gut can lead to a susceptibility to many disorders and diseases of the body. If optimal nutrition is not maintained, food intake can become further decreased and bacterial populations in the bowel change. In this circumstance, there is a shift away from the presence of friendly bacteria. This whole situation is another example of a viscous cycle of "ill health" that can be broken by probiotic therapy (feeding friendly bacteria).

Many pet owners seek "peak performance living" for their loved companions. For the owner of a "competitive animal" (pet), peak performance is very important. Many pets love competition and We are great supporters of "ethical", competitive sports with animals. It may come as a pleasant surprise to pet owners (and some veterinarians) that probiotics have been shown to increase overall performance in competitive animals. Carefully controlled research studies have shown the ability of probiotics to improve performance in competitive horses. We have good reason to suspect that the beneficial effects of probiotics are shared by dogs, cats and humans.

Dr. T. Art (1994) checked cardiac, respiratory, general body chemistry and blood function in competitive racehorses after they had been given probiotics. Overall, measurable improvements in performance were apparent in this important study (Vet Res, 251:361,1994). In particular, desired improvements in aerobic metabolism (body chemistry during exercise) were noted in these studies. Probiotics seem to have a role in optimizing health as well as preventing or treating many diseases. Thus, probiotics contribute to "peak performance".

Probiotics fight unfriendly microbes and toxins

Probiotic therapy can viewed as a circumstance of "microbes" (friendly bacteria) fighting "microbes" (unfriendly yeast, viruses and bacteria). It is a natural extension of current medical research to use friendly bacteria in other ways. Friendly bacteria can be used to clean up the environment, promote the health or growth of plants and they are applied in the modern art of genetic engineering. For example, certain bacteria can be used in contaminated landscapes to degrade toxic solvents that have been used in chemical engineering. The facilitation of the growth of certain bacteria in garbage dumps can result in accelerated decomposition of organic matter. Microbes compete with other microbes, and in the case of the bowel, the seeding of friendly bacteria appears to hold much promise for optimum well-being.

Prebiosis: Feeding the friendly bacteria their own food

There are certain components of a pet's diet that will tend to promote the growth of friendly bacteria and others that do the opposite. Extensive research has shown that giving friendly bacteria (the act of probiotic therapy), with the food that the friendly bacteria live on (prebiosis), improves their chance of colonizing the bowel. It is one thing giving the oral friendly bacteria, but it is another to have them implant and grow in the bowel. Their implantation and growth is assisted by giving their desired food substrate. Giving food for friendly bacteria to implant, grow and live on is called "prebiosis".

The most popular, tried and trusted bacterium for probiosis is the organism Lactobacillus acidophilus. Ideal probiotic products contain prebiotics (food), and in the case of Lactobacillus species, "big sugars" called fructooligosaccharides (or FOS) are highly valuable prebiotics. This is why our recommendations include FOS (Table 21). These big sugars (FOS) do occur naturally. For example, they are found in bananas and onions - foods that are not often given to our pets.

Ingredients	Amount
Protease 18M u/g	5 mg
Amylase 18M u/g	5 mg
Lipase 5M u/g	5 mg
Cellulase 10M u/g	5 mg
Lactase 1M u/g	5 mg
Bromelain	5 mg
Pepsin	2.5 mg
Papain	5 mg
L. Acidophilus 4 billion/g	50 mg
Milk Thistle 40% Extract	100 mg
Brewers Yeast	2487.5 mg
Cranberry	2.5 g
Garlic	100 g
Spinach	100 mg
Fructoligosaccharides	100 mg

Table 21

The four basic factors involved in balancing digestive health are: 1. Probiotic therapy. This proposed digestive food supplement contains a viable, implantable, ideal strain of Lactobacillus acidophilus, which is the most revered probiotic organism. 2. Prebiotic therapy. Fructooligosaccharides facilitate the growth and implantation of Lactobacillus acidophilus. 3. Digestive enzymes are very important for the efficient utilization of food during digestion. 4. Detoxification is a very important component, linked to digestive health. Milk thistle assists liver detoxification. In addition, our recommendations includes the benefits of cranberry, garlic, spinach and brewers yeast. These are optimal sources of several vital nutrients and minerals.

Digestive Enzymes

Food enzyme nutrition is a very important emerging concept in holistic veterinary medicine (and human medicine). Without an adequate supply of digestive enzymes, food cannot be utilized by the body and illness is inevitable. There are many situations that are described in holistic animal care where enzyme supplements in the diet may improve pet well-being and health.

A number of types of enzymes act to break down various food components in the digestive tract. These digestive enzymes differ generally from the metabolic enzymes that occur in cells and body tissues. Enzymes play a pivotal role in healthy chemistry of the body. Digestive enzymes are produced by the salivary glands for action in the mouth. The stomach secretes acid and the enzyme pepsin, which partially digests protein. The pancreas gland has enzymes that act in the small bowel (on proteins and fats) and the walls of the small intestine have their own enzymes.

Each digestive enzyme tends to be quite specific in its effects. Some enzymes breakdown proteins (proteases), some breakdown fats (lipases) and many breakdown sugars (amylase and disaccharidases, such as lactase). Please note that the substrate (food component) upon which the enzyme acts, e.g. the sugar lactose, is changed by one letter to label the enzyme – i.e. lactose is digested by lactase. Thus, the substitution of key letters in the name of the food with the letter a often comes up with the name of the food (e.g. cellulose digested by cellulase, lipid by lipase, protein by protease etc.). Valuable digestive supplements are formulated with a complete array of digestive enzymes (Table 21).

Situations where digestive enzymes are often required

General illness, stress of any kind, food intolerance or allergy and drug treatments have all been implicated in situations where digestive enzymes are not secreted in optimal amounts by the gastrointestinal tract. In these situations, enzyme production is often insufficient, food is not adequately absorbed and nutrition becomes sub-optimal. On the other hand, studies in veterinary medicine show that the use of certain digestive enzymes as supplements can improve the efficiency of animal feeding.

Although further studies on the health benefits of digestive enzyme supplements in dogs, cats and horses are required, much evidence exists to define their beneficial effects. Certain enzymes (papain from papaya and bromelain from pineapples) have been described as having a "pain relieving" effects following exercise. Many studies point to the benefit of using bromelain (extract of pineapples) for improving rehabilitation from soft tissue injuries (see section 2, Bone and Joint Health). Active animals are always producing minor injuries to their soft tissues.

Enzyme supplements are believed to play a special role in cancer or states of immunodeficiency. For example, bromelain may inhibit the spread (metastasis) of certain types of cancer and some enzymes have been used as support for immune function in cancer and AIDS (or animal equivalents e.g. immunodeficiency provoking viruses in dogs and cats). By mechanisms unknown, the enzyme papain (found in papaya) may be a potent pain-killing agent that suppresses inflammation. Some studies have suggested that papain may be as effective as aspirin in some pain control studies in animals.

The most underestimated area for the application of digestive enzymes in pets is in the care of elderly cats, dogs and horses. Digestive functions tend to be compromised with age and digestive enzyme supplements are especially important for the "geriatric" pet or human. Furthermore, any physical or mental stress from many disorders may benefit from digestive enzyme supplementation, in order to create optimal circumstances for good nutritional status.

Detoxification

The process of "body cleansing" and the removal of toxins (detoxification) is very popular in human, eclectic, medical practice. Detoxification is now a major issue in holistic medical care for pets and humans. Our pets (like us) are constantly exposed to environmental toxins and some toxins are generated in the bowel itself. The generation of bowel toxins can be variably prevented by probiotic treatments that are ideally combined with prebiosis (food for friendly bacteria see Table 22). Environmental toxins include food additives, household poisons (e.g. cleaning agents), pesticides, herbicides and even shampoos or pet cosmetics.

The body has an elaborate series of working, chemical systems that result in detoxification (the elimination of toxins from the body). Regularity of bowel and urinary function is necessary for the body to remain free of toxins. Clearly, the avoidance of toxin exposure is the primary issue, but toxin avoidance in our modern environment is impossible. Several organs in the body play a key role in eliminating toxins but the liver is the dominant organ of detoxification.

The liver engages in elaborate chemistry to detoxify and change toxins into chemicals that can be excreted from the body by the kidneys and in the stool (via bile secretions). Regularity of bowel habit in pets is important in the act of whole body detoxification. Again, probiotics are quite helpful because they will tend to promote optimal digestive function and stooling, as well as acting as detoxifying agents within the bowel itself.

Toxin accumulation in the body has been linked to the occurrence of a wide range of diseases including cancer, arthritis, immune disorders and behavioral problems in pets (and humans). The subject of detoxification of chemicals by the liver is extraordinarily complex. The liver acts like a factory and processing plant. Without the liver's ability to efficiently process toxins, chronic disease often emerges. The liver requires many nutrients and antioxidants to go about its work, but certain herbal agents have been found to be particularly valuable in assisting the process of detoxification by the liver. Of all proposed detoxifying herbs, milk thistle (Silybum marianum, containing silymarin) appears to be of particular benefit to the liver.

Milk thistle - A special "detoxifying" herb

Milk thistle contains natural chemicals called flavones (sily-marin) that have been shown in several scientific studies to both assist in the process of detoxification by the liver and exert a protective effect on the liver against damage from toxins. Milk thistle appears to prevent the depletion of a small peptide (protein) called glutathione. Glutathione is required for detoxification processes in the liver and it is found to be depleted in several diseases e.g. immune deficiencies, liver disease and lung disease. Several other herbs with antioxidant properties have been used to assist in detoxification process, but milk thistle seems to have special properties. The use of milk thistle has far reaching potential for pet's health by its assistance in the everyday activities of detoxifying many of the common toxins that our pets are exposed to on a daily basis.

The Four Principles of Healthy Digestive Function

It can be seen that the four areas of important support of digestive functions are:

1. Probiotic therapy: the administration (feeding) of friendly bacteria, especially Lactobacillus acidophilus.

2. Prebiotic therapy the administration of food that supports the growth of friendly bacteria, especially fructooligosaccharides (FOS).

3. Digestive enzymes: the administration of a variety of enzymes that help the assimilation of nutrients by the body. Enzymes can help assist in the digestion of protein, fats, carbohydrates and certain kinds of fiber.

4. Detoxification: the process of avoiding toxins from the bowel and helping the main organs of the body (especially the liver) to eliminate toxins. The herb milk thistle plays a special role in supporting the detoxifying functions of the liver.

These four areas of pivotal support for digestive health are a particular focus of holistic veterinary care. These concepts have been identified and used to develop holistic digestive supports by holistic vets (Table 21).

Combining the four principles of digestive health for pets

Dietary supplements can be available in convenient powder formats that combines probiosis, prebiosis, digestive enzymes and detoxification. A formula is listed in Table 21. The chosen probiotic is a viable strain of Lactobacillus acidophilus which is supported by the prebiotic actions of fructoligosaccharides (FOS). The proposed formula contains a wide array of digestive enzymes including: protease, lipase, amylase, lactase and cellulase to assist in rendering food ready for absorption into the body.

The presence of milk thistle in digestive nutraceuticals has beneficial actions on the function of the liver and it supports the body's' systems of detoxification. In order to render the digestive mix palatable and to supply many nutrient co-factors, a generous portion of brewer's yeast can be added. Brewer's yeast provides a whole host of essential amino acids, vitamins and trace minerals (see section 2. In addition, dried yeast is rich in beta glucan, an agent that has potent benefits of stimulating immune functions in the body (section 2). Readers are encouraged to speak to their vets.

Summary

Digestive function is highly complex. The most important aspect of its function involves the maintenance of healthy contents of the gut (good diet and friendly bacteria) and the enzymatic digestion of food components (digestive enzymes). The combination of probiosis, prebiosis, digestive enzymes and detoxifying herbs is an optimal approach to help promote healthy digestive function (Tables 20 and 21). Many products are available that select one or two of these approaches e.g. probiosis alone, "detox" alone etc. However, a complete, combined approach for a natural way to digestive health involves all these approaches. A holistic combination of agents for support of digestive function, is more cost-effective. Without a healthy digestive tract, a pet's general health will undoubtedly suffer, ask your vet.

Immune Health: The Omega and Immune Factor

Getting to know immune function

The immune system is ever vigilant in protecting the body from infections and disease. Immunity can sometimes be weak (immune deficiency) or it can go haywire and attack the body itself (autoimmunity). The immune system is composed of many specialized types of white cells, which can engulf foreign particles (antigens engulfed by macrophages); or it can produce antibodies (B lymphocytes); or it can directly attack antigens (T lymphocytes). The main functions of T and B cells and consequences of their deficiency are summarized in Table 22. The organs of the immune system are composed in part of collections of these immune competent cells. The immune organs include lymph nodes, the spleen and the thymus gland.

The complex immune system is under constant exposure to toxins or infectious agents like bacteria, viruses, yeasts and parasites. In order to function, it requires special nutritional support and general "nurturing". This section will focus on nutrients that are particularly valuable for supporting the immune system. However, the correct balance of immunity and its role in preventing disease is highly complicated.

Comprehensive discussions of immunity involve issues such as correct vaccination of pets and specific therapies that combat infection e.g. antibiotics. Also, the immune system has complex ways of communicating within itself and with the rest of the body. It is highly regulated and influenced by many factors including: the presence of disease, stress and, of course, optimal nutrition. The immune system participates very closely in allergic reactions, all types of inflammatory disease and the maintenance of general health.

B-cell deficiencies	T-cell deficiencies
Recurrent respiratory infections	Gut candidiasis
Bacterial infections, local sepsis, meningitis	Opportunistic infections e.g. mycobacteria, pneumocystis
Reduced lymph node mass	Recrudescent viral infections e.g. Herpes, shingles
Frequent digestive disorders with diarrhea and malabsorption	Wasting, failure to thrive in children and digestive disorders
Emergence of autoimmune disorders Skin disorders	Graft versus host disease Skin disorders. Loss of thymic function
Blood disorders, hemolytic anemia, neutropenia, low platelet counts	Blood changes e.g. eosinophilia

Table 22
Features associated with B or T cell deficiencies. Some disorders are common to both. Deficiencies can occur together.

The importance of optimum intake of omega 3 fatty acids for health has resulted in the preparation of many foods that are fortified with these types of fats. However, it must be understood that the "active" forms of these omega 3 fatty acids are the ideal way of obtaining the "active" types of fatty acids. The active forms are conveniently available in fish oil. In the case of pets, the fish oils can be given in convenient, stabilized, fish oil powders.

Immune supporting nutrients

The sophisticated functions of the immune system require a vast array of vital nutrients. Almost every essential nutrient, vitamin and trace elements is involved directly or indirectly in immune mechanisms. However, certain nutrients play a special role in promoting healthy immunity. These include essential fatty acids especially of the omega 3 type (found in fish oil), vitamin C, the metal zinc and the complex of B vitamins. In addition, there are many naturally occurring substances that can help to boost immunity. A good example is beta glucan that is found in high concentrations in Brewer's yeast (see sections 2 and 6). It is important to review several these principal immune balancing or immune boosting nutrients. For a fuller account of this subject by the author, readers are referred to the book "Natural Ways to Healthy Immune Function" (by S. Holt, www.wellnesspublishing.com).

The Omega Immune Factors

Pet owners have heard a lot about "good fats" and "bad fats" in the diet of humans and animals (see section 3). Dogs and cats lean towards a carnivorous diet, whereas horses are vegetarian. Thus, there is a lot of wisdom in the statement "horses for courses". There is no doubt that excessive saturated fat intake is not as damaging to a dog as it is to a human. Excessive saturated fat (bad fat) intake in humans is clearly linked to heart disease and cancer (see Natural Ways to a Healthy Heart, by Holt S, M. Evans Publishers Inc., 1999), but this may not be the case in all pets.

In an oversimplified way, we now talk about good fats, some of which are absolutely "essential". The word "essential" implies that they have to be present in the diet in correct forms and amounts. This is why these liquid types of fat are called essential fatty acids. These essential fatty acids are liquid because they are chemically unsaturated, in contrast to solid fat that is saturated (with hydrogen). Essential fats are very important for cellular health. They aggregate to form the membranes around cells.

The detailed chemistry of fats is not as important as understanding their functions. To reiterate, essential fatty acids are labeled "essential" because they cannot be synthesized in humans and several animal species. There are two main types of essential fatty acids that are discussed in modern, pet nutrition. These matters were reviewed in sections 3 and 5 but they are so important that they deserve further discussion. In humans, the principle types of "good fats" are examples of omega 6 types of fatty acids and the second are the omega 3 types of fatty acids. Omega 3 types of fatty acids are most often found in fish or marine mammals, whereas omega 6 types of fatty acids are found in the diet in vegetable oils. Omega 6 fatty acids are generally quite available in many pets' diets. It is the omega 3 types of fatty acids that are very important for health in pets and humans. Evidence exists that there is a common and widespread deficiency of omega 3 fats in the diets of humans and pets.

Although "precursors" of omega 3 fatty acids are found in some plants, e.g. flax or soy oils, these precursors are not always converted to the active forms of omega 3 fatty acids, notably EPA (eicosapentanoic acid) and DHA (docosahexanoic acid). Deficiency of omega 3 fatty acids in pets' diets has been described as an important, often missing, health link in nutrition. Why?

The omega 3 factor and health

There are many effects of essential fatty acids. They control the production of vital "hormone – like" substances in the body called "prostaglandins". These prostaglandins are produced in balanced amounts from essential fatty acids and they are involved in many body functions (Table 14.)Upsetting the balance of essential fatty acids upsets many body functions (Table 15.) In general, the ratio of omega 6 to omega 3 fatty acids seems important in this balance and there is a common problem with deficiency of omega 3 fatty acids in pets and humans (Table 23). This means that the ratio of omega 6 to omega 3 fatty acids is often disturbed because of a relative deficiency of the omega 3 types (Table 23).

OMEGA-6 FATTY ACIDS MAY BE OVERABUNDANT IN SOME DIETS

Family	Omega-3 Fatty Acids	Omega-6 Fatty Acids
Principal precursors found mainly in vegetables	Linolenic acid (omega-3)	Linoleic acid (omega-6)
Fatty acid derivatives found mainly in animals (6) or fish (3)	DHA, EPA	GLA, DGLA, and arachidonic acid
Prostaglandins		Type 3 and less Type 2 and leukotrienes inflammatory leukotrienes

Table 23
The role of omega-3 and omega-6 fatty acids as precursors of compounds that are necessary for healthy body functions.

The issue of stabilization of EPA and DHA in fish oil is very important when it comes to active omega 3 fatty acids. These acids, EPA and DHA, can become rancid (oxidized) very quickly and they must be stabilized (Table 24).

Ingredients	Amounts
Powdered omega 3 fatty acids	0.7 g
Flax seed powder	0.1 g
Rice bran powder	0.05 g
Brewers yeast	0.05 g
Wheat germ powder	0.1 g

Table 24
The holistic formulation of an immune supporting supplement.

How does the omega factor operate?

The role of omega 3 fatty acids (fish oil, EPA, DHA) in health maintenance is well established but their mechanism of action is quite complex. Omega 3 fatty acids are part of all cell membranes and they are responsible for basic cellular health in all body tissues. They play as special part in keeping the skin moist and supple (hydrated) and they are an absolute prerequisite for healthy coat and skin in pets (see section 3). The omega 3 fats (EPA and DHA) are found in high concentrations in the brain and nervous system (see section 5). They are very important in brain development in pets and recent research shows that they can affect behavior (section 5). Fish oil (EPA and DHA) has antidepressant actions that have been well demonstrated in several human studies. In addition they are believed to be beneficial in humans in attention deficit disorder (ADD) and neurological illnesses, such as multiple sclerosis.

Omega 3 fats are important for immune function but they exert special anti-inflammatory effects by their actions on "balancing" the production of prostaglandins (Table 23). Studies in animals and humans show that fish oil is a powerful, natural anti-inflammatory agent. It has been used successfully in the treatment of inflammatory bowel disease, asthma and rheumatoid arthritis. This anti-inflammatory effect of fish oil is due mainly to the balance of the production of prostaglandins. Fish oil favors the production of anti-inflammatory, "tissue stabilizing", prostaglandins. Clearly, it is apparent that the description of omega 3 fatty acids from fish oil as an important nutritional link to health is well justified. Omega 3 fatty acids (DHA and EPA) have potent and versatile health giving benefit for pets.

The holistic nature of the Omega Immune Factor

Given the recent interest in the maintenance of optimal immunity, a number of natural products have been produced to boost or balance immunity. The idea of boosting immunity, without due attention to balance, is naïve. Whilst immunodeficiency can be a big problem in pets, the immune system is sometimes quite aggressive and uncontrolled. For example, with increasing age, there is a tendency for the body to attack itself somewhat (autoimmunity). Thus, the components of aging immunity (immune senescence) are a complex mixture of immune deficiency in the presence of a variable degree of "self-attack" (autoimmunity). These concepts are simplified. For readers interested in a more detailed discussion of the functions of the immune system and its regulation by natural remedies, the book "Natural Ways to Healthy Immune Function" (Holt S., www.wellpublishing.com) is recommended.

The Omega Factor is a holistic mixture of nutrients that are known to contain agents that will support healthy immune function. It avoids the inclusion of specific, potent immune stimulators, which can be used independently, as required. The Omega Factor contains generous amounts of omega 3 fatty acids that are balanced with a content of omega 6 fatty acids in an approximate ratio of 3:1. It contains beta glucan, which is known to stimulate immunity by actions on specific types of white cells in the immune system. Beta glucan has become very popular as an immune stimulant and it is present in Brewers yeast. Flax seed and wheat germ powder provide an essential array of vitamins and minerals that complement the important nutrients found in Brewers yeast. Rice bran powder has been identified as an agent that can also stimulate white cell function through its content of polysaccharides.

Beta glucan

Beta glucan is a complex polysaccharide (big sugar) that is found predominantly in the yeast (Saccharomyces cerevisiae), cereal grains (oats and barley) and many medicinal mushrooms. Its chemical structure resembles the "glucans" that have been isolated from medicinal mushrooms and studied for their health benefits. Beta glucan has been used in alternative medical practice to enhance immune function, promote wound healing and lower blood cholesterol.

There are polysaccharide receptors on certain immune competent cells and it is believed that this polysaccharide (beta glucan) stimulates or "primes" their activity. All glucans are made up of simple sugars (e.g. glucose) linked together in various chemical configurations. Glucans from different sources tend to have a different linkage pattern of simple sugars. For example, yeast derived glucan is a 1,3/1,6 linked molecule, whereas the glucan from maitake mushroom has a reverse in this chemical configuration.

In the early 1980's, Dr. J.K. Czap and K. F. Austen defined

the presence of a receptor for beta glucan on human monocytes and studied its actions (J. Immunol, 134, 2588-93, 1985). When beta glucan binds to the macrophage (monocyte) receptor it induces several functional changes. The macrophage tends to increase its phagocytic ability (c.f. Echinacea) and release several cytokines (e.g. IL-1 and -2). This triggers other cells, such as T lymphocytes, to exert their function. One added mechanism of action of beta glucan is believed to be a significant antioxidant effect.

There have been several studies with beta glucan in animals and humans that show a clear benefit of this polysaccaride on balancing or stimulating immune functions. For example, in one study, the feeding a yeast-derived supplement containing beta glucan to victims of severe trauma resulted in a six-fold reduction of hospital acquired pneumonia. Several uncontrolled, clinical observations suggest that beta glucan may be a valuable cough and cold (flu) preventive and it may have a beneficial effect on wound healing, by presumed immune modulating mechanisms.

There are several new sources of yeast derived beta glucan and not all can be anticipated to have the same biological effects. Betaglucans are an interesting byproduct of yeast fermentation processes and several healthy soybean products are valuable sources of betaglucan, as well as being a source of the health giving fractions of soya beans.

Beta glucan (technical considerations)

Macrophage activation with beta 1-3 glucan is well described in the scientific literature. When macrophages are activated a whole series of chemical events occur with the production of many immune signaling factors (cytokines). Some comparisons of the macrophage stimulating activity of beta glucan from yeast have been made with the polysaccharides (mannans or polymannose) found in Aloe. In general, beta glucan appears to have a greater immune stimulatory action than polysaccharides from Aloe. The potent stimulating effect of beta glucan is believed to be related to the presence of macrophage cell membrane receptors, which are stimulated with its administration. It is proposed that beta glucan is the most ubiquitous macrophage-activating factor found in nature.

Reductions in macrophage function occur as a consequence of exposure to immunotoxins, stress and overwhelming infections.

Yeast derived beta 1-3 glucan has been proposed as an effective way of countering these non-specific immune deficiencies. Beta glucan has been shown to play a role in the release of IL-1 and IL-2 (cytokines), the stimulation of bone marrow function and T cell activation. Protagonists of the therapeutic use of beta glucan have proposed beneficial effects in HIV disease, many conditions which cause oxidative stress (e.g. heavy exercises) and as a prophylaxis against respiratory infections. It may have special role in the treatment of arteriosclerosis. In this latter circumstance, the activation of macrophages may play a role in decreasing plaque formation in arterial blood vessels. The antioxidant actions of beta glucan found in Brewer's yeast are very valuable.

Summary

In brief, the interconnections of the immune system with many body functions means that optimal immunity is an absolute prerequisite for good health. In general terms, the Omega 3 fatty acids and other nutrients can be seen to support general health with value for cardiovascular, joint and brain function. It is an important and vital source of essential nutrients that may be missing in the diet of many dogs, cats or horses. It provides an essential health link, especially due to its provision of essential fatty acids of the omega 3 type.

**LOVE YOUR PET AND
VISIT YOUR VET**

Ear Health

Checking your pets ears

Ear problems are one of the commonest causes of pet discomfort, but they are often forgotten by pet owners. Every few days, pets' ears should be checked for signs of abnormality. It is often a mistake to seek meticulous appearance of pets' ears by frequent cleaning. An animal produces a small amount of wax and superficial sebaceous secretion to maintain ear health. For example, the repeated application of drying agents or soap can cause ear inflammations and eczema.

Often the signs of ear problems are not obvious. A common sign of ear discomfort is head shaking and sometimes self-destructive behavior may occur. Excessive paw chewing or general bad behavior should prompt a quick look at the ears.

Most ear problems are minor, but the ear is a sensitive organ that is easily damaged. Examination of ears by the pet owner should be limited to inspection and touching of the external (outside) ear parts. Never poke the ears or push cotton or cue tips into the ear canal of your pet. Serious damage can occur. If your pet has "floppy" ears, problems are quite common. Warm weather brings a greater burden of parasites, fleas, mites and insects for pets. These unwanted guests love the environment of the ear of your pet.

Common ear problems

Common disorders of the ear include mite or flea infestations, infections with fungi or bacteria, minor injury (scratches or small blood blisters) and the lodgement of foreign bodies (e.g. plant parts, soil or excessive dust). If the ears look inflamed or if there is any sign of exudates or pus, a visit to the veterinarian is required.

Recurrent problems with the external ear can occur with poor grooming and following courses of antibiotics that disturb the normal, friendly bacteria in the ear (and the gut). The ears are often involved in general allergies. Holistic veterinarians have stressed the role of probiotic therapy in helping to balance the body following antibiotic treatments and digestive nutraceuticals may help in some circumstances. Deficiencies of immunity can sometimes present as ear problems, e.g. feline leukemia or other causes of immune deficiency.

Cleaning ears

Ears are sensitive and cleaning must be gentle. In the presence of minor irritations or infections of the outer ear, an initial gentle wipe with warm water is required. During cleaning, cats and dogs will invariably try and shake their heads. Let them, this loosens up material that you need to wipe away. It is important not to introduce soap or detergents into the ear canal. These can make irritations worse and they leave an irritating residue on the skin of the outer ears, which can result in eczema or crusting.

The use of botanicals and herbals with oils

There are a number of excellent herbal remedies for common ear problems (Table 25). Herbals can be used to help inhibit infections with bacteria, yeasts and fungi. However, it should be stressed that serious infections, or inner ear problems, cannot be treated by topical agents and the advice of a veterinarian is always required with significant illness.

Ear problems with mites, ticks and fleas can be seasonal, with a preponderance of infections in warm weather. Herbals, botanicals or oils administered in a topical manner may be useful preventives against ear infestations. The problem with simple herbal tinctures (fluids) is that they tend to rapidly drain off the skin, whereas oil-based drops tend to cling to the skin. Oils create a valuable, soothing residue to fight infections and counter excessive drying of the earflaps.

Certain oils of plants have significant antimicrobial actions. In fact, essential oils of plants are responsible for the plant's own resistance to infection in nature. Many herbs and oils have been suggested for their skin-softening, soothing and antimicrobial actions, but of particular value is garlic oil. Many microbes just cannot live in garlic oil – it is one of nature's mixtures of "natural antibiotics".

Simple castor oil is also valuable for breaking up wax concretions and maintaining suppleness of the skin of the external ear.

A proprietary blend of:

Mullein flower
Oregon grape
Garlic oil
Marshmallow
Vitamin E
Oil of Palma Christi
Acetic acid
Boric acid

Table 25
The all-natural contents of a herbal, oil, topical antiseptic. www.naturesbenefit.com

When garlic oil is combined with Mullein flower and Oregon grape a particularly powerful topical "antimicrobial" is produced. Oregon grape contains berberine, which is revered in natural medicine as a key antimicrobial. Herbalists claim that berberine may be more effective than certain antibiotics against specific pathogenic (disease causing) bacteria. It has a wide spectrum of antibacterial activity and it is also antifungal in its actions. Oregon grape alone has been recommended as an effective antimicrobial ear application in an oil base. Its contents are known as the "naturopathic antibiotic". It should be recognized that topical antimicrobials may not be as specific at eradicating certain infections as certain antibiotic drugs.

Mullein flower is a common weed that was imported into the US from Eurasia. The leaves of Mullein have mild astringent properties and they have been widely used as an effective application for minor wounds and scratches. An active pet commonly has minor wounds on his or her ears. Mullein has well described antiviral properties (e.g. herpes simplex virus, HSV), antibacterial properties, antifungal properties and it is known to be effective against mites, fleas and "mange". These properties make Mullein a versatile, antiseptic herbal that is described as having special properties (affinity) against ear infections.

Marshmallow is known for its wide ranging and safe benefits

for pets. It contains "mucilage" that deals with irritations of the skin and abrasions of delicate mucous membranes. Marshmallow is believed to provide a soothing and lubricating barrier over delicate areas of skin and it helps to prevent irritations by noxious agents. When applied to insect stings, bites, scratches and inflammations, marshmallow has both healing and immune stimulating properties. Scientific studies have shown it to be active against several bacteria including bacteria of the genus Staphylococcus, Proteus and Pseudomonas. The bacteria of the genus Pseudomonas can cause chronic, difficult to treat ear infections.

Two simple, but tried and trusted antiseptics are acetic acid (vinegar) and boric acid. Acetic acid alters the acidity (pH) of the external ear and it favors the growth of "friendly" types of bacteria on the external ear.

Natural Approaches

Having accepted the individual benefits of many natural agents for dealing with common problems of the external ear, a rational approach to ear health is a combined herbal and botanical approach (Table 25). The advantages of the prolonged residence time of oil-based drops on the ear are clear. The holistic combination of the many natural substances to promote ear health is found in many holistic veterinarian publications (Table 25).

Summary

Natural approaches to ear comfort can be applied by a simple dropper to the external ear. These oily mixtures cling to the skin of the outer parts of the ear. They have a characteristic odor largely from their content of garlic. They can be used intermittently or continuously when required to maintain health of the outer ear.

DO NOT NEGLECT YOUR PET'S EARS

SECTION 9
Antiangiogenesis

What is angiogenesis?

Angiogenesis (the growth of new blood vessel) is a major component in the development of cancer, arthritis, proliferative vascular disease and common skin disease. The increased understanding of the complex cascade of events in angiogenesis has heralded research on inhibitors or modulators of new blood vessel growth. Several drugs or derivatives of natural substances are in clinical trial as angiogenic promoters or inhibitors to combat cancer, cardiovascular and skin disorders. Cartilage and its extracts have been studied in detail and presented with both scientific excellence and unfortunate "hype". Other natural substances that modulate angiogenesis include various animal or marine biologicals, the soy isoflavone genistein, colostrum and extracts of fungi and plants (e.g. green tea). "Natural" antiangiogenesis (interference with unwanted, new blood vessel growth) has great promise in veterinary practice.

The phenomenon of angiogenesis (new growth of blood vessel, angio=blood vessel, genesis=growth) has attracted considerable interest in the scientific community. Angiogenesis play a major role as a determining factor in a variety of diseases, including: cancer, arthritis, skin conditions, eye disorders, and inflammatory disease. The application of methods to manipulate angiogenesis has created fascinating, complementary, treatment options, including the potential use of natural-based compounds that may modify new blood vessel growth.

Angiogenesis and Disease

Angiogenesis can best be defined by dissecting the world to its Greek roots: "Angio"- and "Genesis". Angio is Greek for "a vessel, usually a blood vessel" and genesis means, "to originate or create." Angiogenesis is thus the growth of new blood vessel, a process that can happen in normal or disease-state circumstances in the tissues of the body. This process is also called neovascularization ("neo" means "new"). The phenomenon of angiogenesis has attracted considerable interest in the scientific community. In the normal adult, angiogenesis occurs infrequently. Exceptions are found in the female reproductive system, where it occurs during the development of follicles during ovulation and in the placenta during pregnancy. These periods of angiogenesis are relatively brief and tightly controlled with regard to the extent of new vessel growth.

Angiogenesis is a multi-step event in which endothelial cells, those that form the walls of small blood vessels (capillaries), migrate (move) and proliferate (divide). The capillary formation is triggered by several agents thought to be released largely from tissues near proliferating capillaries. Substances made in the body, called fibroblast growth factors, and other molecules, have the ability to induce all the steps necessary for angiogenesis.

Normal angiogenesis also occurs as part of the body's repair processes, that is, in the healing of wounds and fractures. Angiogenesis also plays a major role in a variety of diseases, including: cancer (the growth of solid tumors), arthritis, artherosclerosis, skin condition, eye disorders, and inflammatory disease. In these cases, it can often be an unwanted and detrimental phenomenon. By adding the word inhibitors to angiogenesis, we have a descriptive phrase for compounds, which prevent or reduce the growth of new blood vessels (antiangiogenic compounds). The application of methods to manipulate angiogenesis has created much focused research, including the potential of natural-based compounds that may modify new blood vessel growth.

Neovascularization (new blood vessel supply) of developing, repairing, or neoplastic tissues is regulated, at least partially, by a family of proteins which can be extracted from a certain vascular tissue, such as cartilage. These extractable proteins are known by a variety of terms, such as anti-invasion factors (AIV) or angiogenesis inhibitors. They act as local regulators for some of the major mechanisms by which endothelial cells are thought to invade tissues during neovascularization (new blood vessel formation).

Modulating Angiogenesis

The process of forming new blood vessels is essential to tissue repair, ulcer healing, ovulation, and menstruation. Vascularization plays a major role in the propagation of several disease states. Judah Folkman, M.D., the of Children's Hospital, Boston, and Harvard Medical School, is credited with the discovery of importance of angiogenesis in tumor development. His research has offered a unique and promising basis for the therapeutic application of antiangiogenic and proangiogenic compounds. Some natural compounds, such as shark cartilage and soy isoflavones, may modulate angiogenesis in vivo (in the intact animal). Whilst the effects of these natural compounds in intact animals or humans have not been explored extensively, such effects are readily apparent in vitro (in laboratory preparations).

The importance of angiogenesis in the promotion of cancer growth has fueled a considerable amount of research into the control and mechanism of angiogenesis. The growth of most solid tumors depends on the development of a tumor circulation, so it seems logical to inhibit this vascularization, thereby causing the death of neoplasia or limitation of tumor expansion. This is the popular concept of starving "cancer or disease to death". Without a nutrient, blood supply tissues die.

Many substances are now recognized as exerting a modulating (balancing) effect on angiogenesis. The initial crude extract of angiogenic factors isolated from neoplasia by Dr. Folkman were referred to as tumor angiogenesis factors (TAFs). A flurry of research has identified inhibitors of TAF and assisted in the characterization of many agents and cofactors that are required for the modulation of angiogenesis. In brief, a complex host of factors control new blood vessel growth.

The simplest way to explain angiogenesis is to consider a four-step process: (1) the localized erosion of the basement membrane in tissues; (2) the migration of activated endothelial cells promoted by angiogenic factors; (3) endothelial cell proliferation; (4) a complex combination of sustaining influences on the angiogenic process. Angiogenic factors and antiangiogenic compounds may play a role in one or more of these four steps.

The complex steps in the process of angiogenesis and its control provide a multitude of sites for the potential application of antiangiogenic or proangiogenic therapy. The large, ever increasing, number of identified angiogenic factors makes it unlikely that one discrete, antiangiogenic molecule can be used alone as a successful treatment. This reinforces the use of potentially more versatile antiangiogenic agents that may have multiple sites of activity. These agents may be used either alone or in combination with other antiangiogenic compounds of natural origin.

Recent research shows that combinations of antiangiogenic therapies with other anticancer therapies, such as immunotherapy or chemotherapy may be a way of amplifying the killing of cancer cells or dealing with unwanted blood vessel growth in arthritis. Shark cartilage, isoflavones of soybean origin and other natural agents, such as green tea, are candidates for much further investigation as antiangiogenic agents in humans and animals.

Factors Controlling Angiogenesis

New blood vessel growth is normally kept under tight control. This control is exerted by a highly intricate and coordinated production of molecules that both promote and suppress angiogenesis. In brief, the control of angiogenesis is orchestrated by different cell types, molecules or soluble mediators and natural compounds within the supporting matrix of connective tissue.

Certain cytokines, growth factors, matrix proteins and other mediators promote angiogenesis whereas others are angiostatic. Angiostatic agents that are involved in the control of new blood vessel growth include thrombospondin (a matrix protein), retinoids, tissue inhibitors of metalloproteinase, platelet factor 4 and selected growth factors.

We have learned a great deal about the complexity of the cascade of events during new blood vessel formation. To summarize, there is activation of endothelial cells, basement membrane rupture, complex processes of cellular adhesion, cellular migration and proliferation. These events result in the sprouting of new blood vessels from existing vasculature. Of particular importance is the synthesis of basement membranes, which are an essential component of blood vessels. This process is associated with an increase in collagen type

IV. The role of basement membrane synthesis in angiogenesis is so important that it has become a key focus for the development of drugs that can alter this process and suppress angiogenesis.

The body has a natural balance of angio-suppressing and angio-promoting factors. This balance is lost in the presence of unwanted angiogenesis that occurs in a variety of disease states, especially cancer, arthritis and proliferative vascular disorders. It is important to recognize the scope of abnormal angiogenesis in the causation of a wide variety of diseases including, but not limited to: vascular disease, ischemic heart disease, atherosclerosis, wound healing, chronic inflammatory ulcers, maturing burns, peptic ulcer disease, rheumatoid arthritis, gingivitis, psoriasis, chronic variants of eczema, acne rosacea, cancer and their metastases and ocular neovascularization diseases, such as diabetic retinopathy, age related macular degeneration and neovascular glaucoma.

Cartilage Controversy

In the mid 1990's, shark cartilage became the most popular unconventional cancer treatment since the Laetrile controversy of the 1970s. This enthusiasm was manifested by premature reports of the beneficial effects of shark cartilage in cancer therapy (I. William Lane, Ph.D., and Linda Comac, R.N., "Sharks Don't Get Cancer", Avery Publishing Group, 1992). Following major controversies and disciplinary actions by the FTC and the FDA against the illegal act of promoting the sale of shark cartilage as a cancer therapy, interest in shark cartilage as a "general" nutraceutical has waned, inappropriately and tragically.

The opportunistic, commercial organizations that have touted the inappropriately premature, cancer claims have turned out to be the biggest enemy against the appropriate use and future research of shark cartilage. However, scientifically appropriate studies are under way to investigate the potential safety and efficacy of cartilage for the treatment of cancer and other chronic diseases that depend on angiogenesis. Controlled clinical trials of extracts of shark cartilage for cancer therapy are being undertaken currently at MD Anderson Cancer Center, The Cleveland Clinic, The Mayo Clinic and other centers, sponsored and overviewed by the National Institutes of Health. Some commercial companies are heavily engaged in further research on the use of shark cartilage and its extracts in topical and systemic therapy.

Illogical projections, scientific naïveté, and commercial interests in shark cartilage have led to an antagonistic division between basic scientists pursuing the mechanisms of angiogenesis and individuals who are enthusiastic about the clinical uses of natural products with angiogenic properties. The danger of the previous "hype" about shark cartilage is that the potential benefits of cartilage and other natural-based-antiangiogenic compounds in certain diseases may be either minimized or overemphasized. In the author's opinion, research on the use of natural-based-antiangiogenic compounds is long overdue, poorly funded, and often forgotten because of the difficulties in protecting nonproprietary treatments. The manufacturers of "nutraceuticals" with antiangiogenic potential have an obligation to fund such research, especially if products are going to be promoted or used for assumed antiangiogenic properties.

Historical Perspective: Cartilage and Antiangiogenesis

To understand the development of the prevailing theory of antiangiogenic therapy with cartilage, one needs to put angiogenesis into historical perspective. The term angiogenesis was coined approximately 60 years ago. In the 1960s and 1970s, experimental animal models were designed to study tumor growth and the importance of neovascularization (new blood vessel supply) as a rate-limiting step in tumor growth was identified.

Several articles in the lay press have traced the history of the early rejection of Dr. Folkman's theories of angiogenesis by the scientific community and their current acceptance, together with an account of his "vindication". A writer for the Boston Globe newspaper (1997) states: *"Dr. Judah Folkman's work illustrates the slow pace of progress in cancer research but his visionary ideas have led to new ways of understanding this pernicious disease and to renewed hope that it can be vanquished".*

The emergence of interest in shark cartilage as a source of angiogenic inhibitors came out of the observations of Drs. Lee and Langer, who trained with Dr. Folkman. They discovered a substance in bovine cartilage with potent angiogenic properties, but recognized that cartilage is present in only relatively small quantities in mammals. Drs. Lee and Langer noted that the shark's skeleton was composed entirely of cartilage and focused on the knowledge that cartilage does not have a network of blood vessels.

There are several protein fractions in shark cartilage that prevent angiogenesis. Crude extracts of shark cartilage have been shown to strongly inhibit tumor-induced neovascularization, whereas bovine cartilage has to be purified by chromatography before angiogenic activity becomes apparent. Recently, patents have been filed on various fractions of the protein content of shark cartilage for their inhibitory effects on angiogenesis. Drs. Lee and Langer (1983) estimated that sharks might contain about 100,000 times more potential antiangiogenic activity per animal than cattle. These observations are some of the compelling reasons to favor shark over bovine or chicken cartilage as a potential natural source of inhibitors of vascularization.

In addition, shark cartilage appears to be nontoxic, even in very large doses. Over many years of research and thousands of human doses, no significant metabolic toxicity has been reported from using shark cartilage that can be ascribed to administering the compound. When administered orally or rectally, shark cartilage has shown no evidence of local or systemic reactions in several clinical trials. The only possible problem is excessive calcium intake when very large doses of cartilage are used in chronic dosing.

The author does not believe that cartilage compounds can be administered rectally as a reliable route for biologically active components of shark cartilage to access the systemic circulation. Injection of crude cartilage in humans and animals presents an antigenic load and is not to be recommended; even though this approach was successfully taken by John Prudden, M.D. of Columbia University, New York. Dr. Prudden used injections of bovine cartilage for disease treatment (arthritis, inflammatory bowel disease, wound healing and cancer).

Use of Antiangiogenic Therapy in Cancer

The rationale for antiangiogenic therapy in neoplastic disease rests upon the hypothesis that tumor growth and metastatic dispersion of malignant disease are angiogenic-dependent processes (depend on new blood vessel growth). In different terms, cancer and other diseases require the development of a blood circulation.

Considerable indirect and direct evidence has accumulated during the past two decades to support this hypothesis and confirm the angiogenic dependence of neoplasia (cancer). The onset of angiogenic activity appears to occur as a definable event in tumor formation, and most tumors progress from a prevascular to a vascular stage. Dr. Folkman's early work showed that a tumor without a blood vessel supply might grow only to a "pin-head" size, whereas growth galloped with a good blood supply, as a consequence of angiogenesis.

A level of antitumor activity of solid dosage formats of shark cartilage has been reported in two small clinical trials, one conduced in Mexico on eight patients and another in Cuba involving about forty patients (Jose Menendez, M.D., and J. Fernandez-Britto, M.D., personal communication, 1994). The Cuban study demonstrated that shark cartilage induced histologic changes in tumors with notable changes in vascular pattern, and these changes were not considered to be explained by chance alone. These observations are significant and need further study.

James Lott, Ph.D., Professor of Physiology and Biophysics at North Texas State University, Denton, Texas, has performed experiments in mice bearing transplanted tumors (data presented at the First International Congress on Alternative and Complementary Medicine, May 1995). After administering shark cartilage, the tumor-bearing mice lived longer and Dr. Lott found definite histologic changes in transplanted tumors that resemble some of the histologic changes observed in tumor specimens examined in the Cuban clinical trial. However, the author has been unable to substantiate any conclusive clinical outcome concerning the benefit of shark cartilage therapy in the Cuban or Mexican studies and Dr. Lott's studies had protocol problems. <u>Any contemporary claims about the benefit of solid dose shark cartilage in the treatment of cancer must be considered to be still somewhat in doubt.</u>

The data from these studies, although subject to contention, provided the rationale for further human testing of shark cartilage in patients with advanced malignancies. Charles Simone, M.D., of the Simone Protective Cancer Institute in New Jersey, received a recommendation from the Office of Alternative Medicine of the National Institutes of Health in the mid 1990's to conduct clinical trials using shark cartilage in advanced cancer, but these studies were placed on hold and Dr. Simone has never published his results in detail. Dr. Simone, however, reported favorable effects of shark cartilage cancer at several scientific meetings. Unfortunately, Dr. Simone's studies may confuse the assessment of shark cartilage as a cancer therapy because his protocol added a ten-point "Anticancer Lifestyle Program" that could have confounded the results. One of the alleged benefits of shark cartilage therapy has been the suggestion that this therapy improves quality of life measures in cancer patients. Therefore, clinical outcomes in studies of shark cartilage need to be clearly identified in clinical protocols.

Shark Cartilage and Cancer

The most significant findings to date in relation to the treatment of cancer with shark cartilage have been reported by researchers at the Cancer Treatment Research Foundation (in cooperation with the Cancer Treatment Centers of America). This study attempted to assess the safety and efficacy of shark cartilage in the treatment of advanced cancer of various types (breast, colon, lung, and prostate) in more than fifty patients. Dr. Dennis Miller presented the results of the trial at the Thirty-third Annual Meeting of the American Society of Clinical Oncology in Denver in May 1997. Overall, shark cartilage exerted no measurable benefit in the treatment of cancer, in this "Miller Study", as measured by lack of a reduction in tumor size or significant improvement in measures of quality of life in the recipients of the shark cartilage therapy. Two patients, however, showed improvement in quality of life as measured by a quantitative scale. Disease stabilization was noted in one in five patients, but the trial supervisor, Dr. Miller, was guarded in his interpretation of the significance of this potentially beneficial effect.

The authors believe that Dr. Miller and others were too guarded in their conclusions and his colleagues could have seriously underestimated the significance of the one in five (20%) disease stabilization in terminal cancer patients in this study. It is notable that these patients had failed all previous therapies. A further Phase II trial of shark cartilage in cancer was conducted by Dr. M. Rothkopf and Drs. Leitner at St. Barnabas Hospital in New Jersey, which also failed to show significant benefit.

All the patients in the "Miller study" had advanced cancer and were terminal and it could be argued that the protocol was not fair appraisal of the treatment. The odds may have been stacked against showing "degrees" of benefit. In addition, the effect of pretreatment on the outcome of shark cartilage therapy could not be assessed. It should be noted that in all trials to date, shark cartilage has been used only in patients who have failed all acceptable cancer therapy and in some who have subsequently failed other alternative medical options.

Although at first sight the results of both of these controlled, open-label observations of shark cartilage as a cancer cure are disappointing. The author and others believe that the observations of disease stabilization in the Miller study are worthy of careful scrutiny and follow-up. Shark cartilage extracts with antiangiogenic activity should not be dismissed as a promising potential cancer therapy. They should be subjected to much further research. Bear in mind, solid dose shark cartilage was used in these studies and not the biologically active fractions of shark that have been isolated and presented in water-soluble or liposome shelf stable emulsions.

Negative Clinical Trials With Shark Cartilage for Cancer

In brief, the researchers in the aforementioned cancer studies *reached negative conclusions* in the face of reporting disease stabilization in approximately one in five patients. There is no question whatsoever that the Miller Study (Cancer Treatment Centers of America Inc.) and the Leitner - Rothkopf Study (St. Barnabas Hospital) cannot be considered a fair appraisal of the ability (or lack thereof) of shark cartilage to benefit cancer patients. Added to this picture are the negative results of very limited studies of shark cartilage therapy, using solid dosing, performed by Dr. Rosenbluth and his colleagues at Hackensack University Medical Center in New Jersey.

New studies are underway using both solid dose shark material and hydorsoluble extracts of shark in larger numbers of patients. One problem is the number of patients required in a prospective study in order to evaluate outcome. Despite the continuing controversy, there are a significant number of commercial companies, scientists, patients and practicing physicians who strongly support the promise of shark cartilage for cancer and other disease treatment.

Clinical Trials of Other Antiangiogenic Modalities

Increasing knowledge of the factors that "switch on" angiogenesis and the "upregulation" of positive angiogenic stimulators has led to several phase I and phase II clinical trials of a variety of antiangiogenic therapies besides cartilage. Trials of the potent antiangiogenic compound pentosan polysulfate have shown some benefit. This is one of a group of polysaccharides that are capable of interfering with the function of heparin-binding growth factors that promote angiogenesis. Other antiangiogenic compounds in clinical trials include alpha interferon, platelet factor IV, and AGM 1470. At least twenty angiogenic agents are in early clinical trials, with some impressions of benefit emerging from these pilot studies.

Not enough attention has been focused on the modulators of angiogenesis from natural sources. Several such compounds have been discovered in addition to those in cartilage. One of the potential angiogenesis inhibitors isolated from cartilage is a collagenase inhibitor. Other natural antiangiogenic substances include vitamin D3-analogues, fumigallin, herbimycin A, green tea and soy isoflavones.

Isoflavones found in soya beans are very exciting compounds. They have direct tumoricidal properties against several tumor types, and they regulate key enzyme expression, that are pivotal processes involved in tumor growth. Isoflavones are antioxidants and they also play a role in apoptosis (cell death).

The principal soy isoflavones genistein, daidzein and glycetein are very interesting polyphenolic phytochemicals with versatile and potential biological effects. Most research has focused on the properties of genistein, which is known to induce significant antiangiogenic effects in animals. Less well known, is work from researchers at Yale University, which has shown that the soy isoflavones exert antiangiogenic effects in humans.

However, a word of caution is required concerning the use of isoflavones in veterinary practice. Evidence exists that several species of animal, notably felines and some birds (parrots) experience toxicity from chronic isoflavone ingestion. Studies on captive cheetahs in North America zoos reveal sporadic death from soy and isoflavone intake, due to liver failure. Death has also been recorded in parrots. There appears to be great interindividual tolerance for soy isoflavones among certain animal species - a phenomenon not shared by humans and other primates or the dog, cow or pig.

Is (Are) the antiangiogenic factor(s) in shark cartilage absorbed?

Press releases have been issued that shark cartilage in solid dosing is not to be perceived as being of any consistent and reliable benefit for cancer therapy, given the current status of our knowledge. However, many scientists believe that shark cartilage contains substances that are antiangiogenic. These substances can be used in research in cancer or other angiogenic dependent diseases with further knowledge about their characterization and use.

We are impressed by the reports of prolonged survival or stabilization of some cancer patients in anecdotal observations, but *anecdotes do not satisfy our necessary burden of proof.* Although we believe that there is a response in some patients (and so do others), the response is inconsistent, infrequent and unreliable with the use of solid dosage formats of shark cartilage. How are these phenomena explained?

Dr. Holt believes that the answer rests in part in the issue of intestinal permeability and systemic bioavailability of the demonstrated antiangiogenic fractions (proteins) that are found in shark cartilage. Enhanced intestinal mucosal permeability ("leaky gut") is associated with a variety of disease including intestinal mucosal disease, arthritis (rheumatoid disease), psoriasis and, of course, cancer. However, the presence of significant enhanced gut permeability is highly variable - about as variable as alleged "responders" with an angiogenic dependent disease are to solid dose shark cartilage therapy! Bear in mind, that enhanced intestinal mucosal permeability (leaky gut) tends often to be associated with angiogenic dependent disease - perhaps this is more than a coincidence?

Dr. Holt postulates that the variable response of individuals with angiogenic dependent diseases to shark cartilage administration is due to the variable access that antiangiogenic protein may have to the systemic circulation. There are several proteins in hydrosoluble extracts of shark cartilage with variable molecular weights (sizes), some of which may gain access through the gut wall into the body but many of which may not. In addition, antiangiogenic proteins are prone to digestion when given orally. They are proteins, which are split by digestive enzymes. The human gut is impervious to molecules much greater than 50,000 Daltons in size (big molecules) and some of the antiangiogenic proteins in shark exceed this size (molecular weight). Thus, Dr. Holt proposes the following for consideration.

1) The individuals who have stabilized or improved the status of their angiogenic dependent disease with shark cartilage may be those who have a leaky gut that lets in macromolecules or fractions of antiangiogenic protein.

2) Systemic access of the antiangiogenic components of shark cartilage is the rate-limiting factor in achieving any benefit in angiogenic dependent disease.

3) Factors or formulations that enhance the access of antiangiogenic protein fractions of shark cartilage may be valuable e.g. liposomes, but immunological consequences are unknown.

Hydrosoluble fractions of shark cartilage with demonstrable in vitro antiangiogenic activity in both CAM assays (chorio-allantoic membrane of the chick embryo) and bovine endothelial cell proliferation assays. These hydrosoluble extracts have been encapsulated in liposomes for delivery. The liposome is created from an essential fatty acid to create in "microbubble" that may partially protect the proteins in the hydrosoluble fractions of shark cartilage from acid hydrolysis or enzymatic digestion in the gut. In addition liposomes can be shown to cross-epithelial barriers efficiently as "carriers". Whilst complete bioavailability cannot be assured with liposome encapsulated hydrosoluble extracts of shark cartilage - facilitated absorption may occur. These issues are waiting to be tested before firm conclusions can be drawn. There are obvious drawbacks because of the variable efficiency of liposome transfer in the gut, but this approach is novel and exciting.

Perspectives on Angiogenesis Research

The use of agents that modulate angiogenesis marries the nutraceutical, biotechnology and pharmaceutical industries - even though many representatives from these branches of medicine would deny this vehemently! We stress the term modulation and introduce the advantage of natural antiangiogenesis inhibition as very attractive because it is often more gentle and perhaps sometimes safer than using "drugs" or "synthetics", with their very potent actions ("all or none" effects). Potency of angiogenesis inhibition has become a problem in clinical trials with some antiangiogenic agents. These agents are so powerful at inhibiting blood vessel growth that they may precipitate unwanted cardiovascular events, due to interruption of the blood supply to normal tissues. After all, as much as biotechnology dreams about the selective localization of therapeutic agents to diseased tissue, non selective actions of chemotherapy, radiation, drugs and even "targeted" agents have a history of progress that has been plagued by lack of selectivity. Ehrlich's concept of the magic bullet (silver bullet) is still a dream

For these reasons, we see some of the most important advances in angiogenesis research in the field of natural therapies. Farsighted companies have stuck with natural approaches and shark cartilage still stands out, as likely to fulfill its promise, even though some people have inflated the anticancer promise of solid dosage, shark cartilage prematurely with their "illogical leaps of faith".

Arthritis and Angiogenesis

Various types of arthritis may be amenable to therapy with antiangiogenic compounds. Shark cartilage has been well recognized as a versatile nutraceutical and it has been characterized as having a major potential application in the treatment of pain and inflammation associated with arthritis in animal studies. In the 1970's, John Prudden, M.D., and colleagues at the Columbia-Presbyterian Medical Center administered bovine cartilage to humans by both mouth and injection to treat osteoarthritis, rheumatoid arthritis, psoriasis, and regional enteritis with significant treatment benefits. However, this group of investigators did not subscribe to the notion that the observed beneficial effects were caused to a major degree by antiangiogenic activity of cartilage.

Several other researchers have reported a clear association between neovascularization and osteoarthritis, adding weight to the rationale to use cartilage and other antiangiogenic compounds to treat arthritis. Shark cartilage is also a rich source of calcium, which is beneficial for patients with osteoporosis who may require calcium supplementation. It has several other "value added" components (see section 2).

Skin Disorders

Angiogenesis play a major role in several types of skin disease, such as psoriasis and eczema, and it is one of the pivotal steps in wound healing. Bovine cartilage preparations have been shown to have beneficial effects on wound healing, and topical application of shark cartilage has accelerated healing of wounds in some circumstances. The tensile strength of wounds has also been significantly enhances by administering cartilage locally to wounds and burns. Many studies have been conduced as a follow-up to this promising research, but proprietary interests have not permitted widespread publication of this important research. Shark cartilage extracts are a key cosmetic ingredient in anti-aging skin formulae (e.g. Estee Lauder Inc.) and it forms the basis of an FDA approved, burn dressing.

Several clinicians have suggested the use of topical or systemic administration of cartilage, especially shark cartilage, as a potential treatment for such skin diseases as psoriasis, contract dermatitis, eczema, pruritis, angiofibroma, hemangioma, Kaposi's sarcoma, and even burns. Because angiogenesis may play an important role in the pathogenesis of these diseases, they may be amenable to antiangiogenic treatment. However, without controlled studies, the result of such treatments become susceptible to illogical projection and misrepresentation of the potential benefits of antiangiogenic compounds.

Eye Disease

Many eye diseases are associated with angiogenesis, including neovascular glaucoma, diabetic retinopathy, retrolental fibroplasia, and subtypes of macular degeneration. Considerable basic scientific research, as well as anecdotal use of shark cartilage in patients with eye disease, seems to support the need for further human clinical trials. Researchers in Israel reported studies using shark cartilage in the favorable treatment of diabetic retinopathy and neovascular glaucoma, but the work has not been published in detail.

Testing Angiogenesis Promoters and Inhibitors

There have been enormous controversies and complex debates about how angiogenesis and its modulation are best measured. Technology for measuring antiangiogenic potential is sometimes relatively crude or subjective (CAM assay) or it is highly intricate and subject to many variables in interpretation. However, in vitro (laboratory) measures of angiogenesis modulation are not reliable predictors of in vivo effects. The best measures of the biological affect of angiogenesis promoters or inhibitors are in intact animal models or in humans. Arguments about "gold standards" in laboratory research of angiogenic effects are futile. What happens with clinical outcome and vascular effects "in vivo" (in the living body) should be the focus of study.

Conclusion

Angiogenesis has been associated with life-threatening pathologies, such as cancer, and contributes to the pathology of disease, such as arteriosclerosis, psoriasis, and arthritis. New drugs and compounds that inhibit angiogenesis are under intense research and development. Once proper clinical trials are completed, natural antiangiogenic compounds, especially shark cartilage extracts, green tea, mistletoe and isoflavones, may well become the first new class of anticancer compounds and afford great promise for the treatment of arthritis and many other diseases.

NATURAL INHIBITORS OF ANGIOGENESIS CANNOT BE CONSIDERED EFFECTIVE CANCER TREATMENTS WITHOUT MORE RESEARCH.

Colostrum

Understanding colostrum

Colostrum is found in the early secretions of breast milk from a mother; it has been called "life's first food". Bovine colostrum has become a very popular dietary supplement in the US with claims of health benefits that vary in credibility. Unfortunately, the sale of valuable colostrum and its components, such as transfer factors (TF) has been supported by some marketing myths and selections of different colostrum supplements have been driven by some contentious arguments that have nothing to do with science. Despite this marketing "free for all", colostrum has some very valuable uses for health promotion. Colostrum can be perceived as the ultimate chemical dialogue of immunity between a mother and her infant. Colostrum is full of messenger molecules, but these molecules can only exert their benefit if they get into the body (are absorbed). This is the "real" issue to be resolved with colostrum as a therapy.

Is colostrum absorbed?

There is no doubt that the newborn has a "leaky gut" (lets big molecules into the body) and "closure" of this "leakiness" occurs in a variable time frame after birth — usually a few weeks or less. In addition, the newborn's gastrointestinal tract does not create quite as hostile a climate for colostrum as does the adult gut. When given to an adult, the proteins, growth factors and immune signaling molecules (cytokines) in colostrum are likely to be at least partially "chopped up" during digestion and absorbed as small nutrient components. These components do not share the biological activity of the parent "big" molecules. However, the issues are complex.

We have recognized the retention of the ability of the human gut to absorb some "big" molecules in adults and we know that a state of optimal health is required for normal discriminating absorptive functions of the gut. This leads to the logical conclusion that facilitated absorption of colostrum (help with the process of absorption) may be necessary in adults. Such approaches have been taken using liposomes (fat bodies, microbubbles of essential fatty acids), which can be used to coat colostrum and help transfer it across the gut wall.

The transfer of certain big molecules may theoretically cause unwanted immune reactions in the body. Despite this theoretical risk, it is clear that in many circumstances complex tissue extracts (such as thymus extracts) and colostrum of bovine origin have not shown a great propensity to cause allergic reactions. This may not be too surprising if purified fractions are used. After all, tolerance occurs and "cross tolerance" seems to be present when it comes to signaling proteins (molecules of emotion), which have similar structures (antigenic determinants) in many animals. These issues are not completely resolved but they are important.

The controversies surrounding the use of colostrum as an effective "therapy" or dietary supplement to favorably alter body structure and function are mounting. In the middle part of the year 2000, frenetic interest in colostrum supplements in the dietary supplement industry was matched by intense criticism from several sectors of conventional medicine.

Colostrum as a dietary supplement

The possibility of stimulating immune function by natural means is a major focus of current interest among practitioners of both allopathic and complementary medicine. The use of colostrum as a promoter of health and well-being has been recognized for centuries and its use is deeply rooted in the act of "filial piety" in Ancient Chinese Culture. In this act, the nursing mother shares breast milk with her elderly relatives and her child.

The use of natural agents such as immune globulins or other products that are produced by the immune system of mammals has been the focus of much research in recent times. The ideas of providing passive immunity with immune globulin, that is administered by injection, is a well-defined medical intervention for the prevention of viral disease. A common example is the use of gamma globulin for the prevention of hepatitis A virus infection. Other products of the immune system that are candidates for use in medical treatment include interferon and molecules that can transfer "immune phenomena" from a donor to a recipient. An example of this latter process is the use of transfer factor (TF), an agent that can transfer cell-mediated immunity.

It is known that TF is contained within certain blood leuko-cyte fractions and such fractions have been used for the adoptive transfer of antigen-specific, cell-mediated immunity in animals and humans. Antigen-specific TF can also be obtained from colostrum or milk that is secreted by the mammary gland of a mammal that has been exposed to a variety of environmental antigens. In simple terms, TF is a component of colostrum that can promote the com-petence of a T lymphocyte in terms of specific immune reactions to specific antigens. The idea that a fraction of colostrum contains TF that can be administered to transfer cell-mediated immunity is very intriguing given the widespread availability of colostrum of bovine origin and the establishment of techniques for the collection of con-centrates of TF and its purification for use as a dietary supplement.

Immunoglobulins in Cow's Colostrum and Milk

A body of literature has appeared over the past 10 years that suggests that immunoglobulins (IgG) of various types (antibodies) have the potential for the treatment or prevention of infectious diar-rhea in human clinical trials. Several studies have shown the protective effects of antibodies in cow's milk against enteric infection in sev-eral different species of mammal. The use of IgG in colostrum as an immunoprophylactic (prevents infection) or therapeutic agent has been described as a very important issue for the standardiza-tion of colostrum that is used in dietary supplements. For example, high temperature sterilized milk has little if any measurable IgG.

Companies that sell colostrum as a dietary supplement are obligated to provide evidence of the presence of IgG in colostrum, if they are suggesting that their supplement has immune protective or enhancing effects. Few companies that make colostrum have pro-vided evidence that they have retained IgG in their products. To compound the issues, the amount of antibody in colostrum is one thing, but how much of it is absorbed intact is another!

One important determinant of the immunotherapeutic poten-tial of certain types of colostrum is believed to be related to the source of the colostrum. The activity of certain types of colostrum is believed to be in part related to the large donor group of animals used as the source of colostrum. A further important issue is the acquisition of colostrum from pasture-fed animals, who are presumed to be exposed to more antigens (microorganisms) than non-pasture-fed cows. We believe strongly that standards are required in dietary supplements that contain colostrum and that disclosures should be made in product specifications by manufacturers.

What is Transfer Factor (TF)? (technical considerations)

In simple terms, TF is an RNA (ribonucleic acid) peptide that is responsible for the adoptive transfer of antigen-specific cell-mediated immunity in animals or humans. Cell-mediated immunity is a function of T-lymphocytes and it is termed delayed hypersensitivity. TF is capable of transferring cell-mediated immunity to specific antigens between animals. This adoptive transfer of cell-mediated immunity to specific antigens was first discovered by H.S. Lawrence, M.D., in 1949. Dr. Lawrence showed that when products of lymphocytes are taken from an individual who has cell-mediated immunity against Mycobacterium tuberculosis (they have a positive skin test against tuberculin, TB), and donated to a recipient who has no cell-mediated immunity to TB (i.e., has a negative skin test to Mycobacterium tuberculosis), then the skin-test positivity could be transferred to the recipient of the viable lymphocytes and their products.

The real significance of Dr. Lawrence's findings was not recognized for several years. At the time that Dr. Lawrence performed his work on the adoptive transfer of antigen-specific cell-mediated immunity, there was still relatively little known about the importance of lymphocytes in immune function.

Focus on transfer factor as a dietary supplement

Transfer factor derived from human, murine, and bovine sources have been extensively studied. The most accessible source of TF is in the colostrum of breast milk and the most widely available form of TF is derived from cow's milk. Transfer factor is composed of a group of small molecules with molecular weights between 3500 and 6000 Daltons. This size of molecules can be expected to be absorbed by the human small intestine, which is variably penetrated by molecules up to a size of approximately 50,000 Daltons.

It is known that TF is quite stable when stored at low temperature but TF may be heat labile. The exact components and structure of TF remain to be determined but there is general agreement that TF has an oligoribonucleotide-peptide structure.

One of the most interesting aspects of the characterization of polyvalent TF is that it is freely available from colostrum that is collected from dairy cattle. In addition, milk is part of the normal human food chain and, therefore, transfer factor prepared from cow's milk (colostrum) can be made available as a dietary supplement. Whilst it is possible to produce antigen-specific transfer factor in cows, there is potential gain from using polyvalent transfer factor that may be available in bovine colostrum. Its immune value is a consequence of a variety of antigenic stimuli that a dairy cow will experience in its normal lifetime. In addition, TF stimulates immunity in a more general, but nonspecific manner.

Immunotherapeutic potential of transfer factor

Overall, it is apparent that TF may be considered as a valuable option in circumstances where there are defects in cell-mediated immunity. Transfer factor is useful in individuals who have selected defects in cell-mediated immunity. Defects in cell-mediated immunity are the hallmark of AIDS and immunodeficiency states caused by viruses in cats and dogs and these T cell defects may be important in the causation or progression of certain types of cancer.

The therapeutic benefit of TF is debated. Transfer Factor is still considered experimental by many physicians and its use has been restricted to circumstances where conventional medication has failed to produce results. This has led to a circumstance where clinical studies have been performed in patients who have already received medication, which may have compromised immune function. For example, in patients with cancer, in whom TF has been used, there has been a frequent circumstance of irreparable damage to the immune system by the preceding administration of chemotherapy and/or radiation. This situation provides a "set up" for failure of TF and other natural medical options. Unfortunately, natural therapies are usually viewed as "second line" (reserve) treatments and they are often evaluated only in patients who are far advanced in their disease status.

Bovine colostrum has real potential benefits

On one hand, it is clear that antigen-specific TF can be used in selected clinical instances, but there may be benefits of using polyvalent (nonspecific) TF as a dietary supplement. Transfer factor is believed to enhance cell-mediated immunity in a nonspecific manner by a factor of up to 15 percent. Overall, TF seems to act as an immune modulator. When there is "too much" or "too little" in terms of an immunologic response, then TF appears to up-regulate or down-regulate immune functions. Transfer factor is an example of an "adaptogenic" messenger molecule or classic, "biological, response modifier".

It should be recognized that colostrum of a general source, such as regular bovine colostrum, contains a variety of other immune enhancing agents. These agents include growth factors, lysozyme, secretory IgA, complement and other proteins such as lactoferrin. The nonspecific immune enhancing effect of transfer factor can be readily demonstrated in laboratory studies of white cell function.

Exciting information has come from experiments in animals where TF has been used beneficially in several viral diseases, such as Newcastle disease or Meyrick's disease (chronic lymphoma) in chickens and equine encephalitis. Some of the experiments on the use of transfer factor in the treatment of cancer have produced conflicting results. This situation may be due, in part, to uncertainty about the constituents administered or uncertainty about the role of cell-mediated immunity in fighting the spread of certain types of cancer. However, cancer therapy is a very promising area for further research with TF.

Immune factors in bovine colostrum

Several companies have developed dietary supplements that are based on colostrum. Gregory B. Wilson, M.D., and Gary V. Paddock, Ph.D., received a patent (U.S. patent no. 4,816,563) for a process to obtain TF from colostrum and use it for the prevention and treatment of disease. These investigators have described a method for concentrating and sterilizing TF from bovine colostrum. The potency of the concentrate can be determined in an assay described in a patent (U.S. patent no. 4,610,878) that they had filed in 1983. In their patent, these investigators have provided

many examples of the application of TF in the treatment or prevention of infection in animal models and by inference in humans.

Daniel G. Clark, M.D., and Kaye Wyatt have drawn attention
to the potentially versatile and potent health benefits of specially
prepared bovine colostrum, in their book titled "Colostrum, Life's
First Food". These authors have provided very useful anecdotal
accounts of research in the use of colostrum and its fractions in the
therapy of a variety of disorders. They point out the importance of
a variety of potentially health giving components of colostrum including: immunoglobulins, lactoferrin, proline-rich polypeptide, insulin-
like growth factors, transforming growth factors, lactoperoxidases,
xanthine oxidase enzymes, lysozyme, cytokines, interleukin-10, gly-
coproteins, trypsin inhibitors, lymphokines, oligopolysaccarides,
orotic acid, and other immune factors. It is clear that colostrum is
a treasure chest of natural substances, which have important implications for the promotion of immune function and health.

In a recent book entitled "Colostrum: Nature's Gift to the
Immune System", Beth M. Ley traces the knowledge that colostrum
(mother's milk) provides an individualized food that is perfectly
engineered to promote and transfer passive immunity to the infant.
Ms. Ley has alleged evidence that adults with immune deficiency
(e.g., AIDS), cancer, and autoimmune problems (e.g. multiple sclerosis, arthritis, etc.) may benefit from the administration of colostrum.
In particular, benefits are to be expected in the prevention or treatment of opportunistic infections in AIDS, such as diarrhea caused
by Cryptosporidium parvum and pathogenic strains Escherichia coli.
The book by Ms. Ley analyzes some of the prevailing scientific literature that reveals the potential immune enhancing, digestive, anti-
infective, and anti-inflammatory benefits of colostrum.

The potential health giving properties of colostrum seem to
extend beyond immune enhancement by providing benefits to body
builders, athletes, and convalescent patients. The mechanisms
whereby colostrum may speed recovery time from illnesses are not
fully understood, but colostrum is known to contain several natural growth factors.

Processing and source of colostrum

The safety and effectiveness of colostrum will vary in a manner dependent on its source and the manner in which it is processed. Several scientists have drawn attention to the heterogeneity (varied nature) of different types of colostrum and methods for its preparation vary considerably. There are many other components of colostrum that exert diverse biologic actions and these components can be present to a variable degree depending upon processing techniques. It is known that heat can denature components of colostrum.

The cow is essentially a "factory" for producing colostrum and this "factory" should not be contaminated with harmful chemicals or drugs. Therefore, pasture-fed cows that are reared on organic farms are a preferable source of colostrum. A cow is exposed to a vast array of antigens in its natural habitat and this exposure is believed to result in the development of natural immunity that may be passed via colostrum in the process of adoptive transfer of immunity.

Arguments prevail among manufacturers of various types of colostrum about the relative benefit of specific processing techniques, sources of colostrum, and modes of delivery. These companies produce colostrum for use in dietary supplements with various claims about the health-giving constituents of their respective colostrum products. Much of the available colostrum used in dietary supplements in the US is frozen prior to transportation. Frozen products have limitations in the manner in which they can be processed and they may not be water soluble or readily dispersible. The most promising delivery of colostrum is in liposomes (fat bodies) that can potentially protect colostrum from complete digestion and help its absorption into the body (Liposome Colostrum).

HOW MUCH COLOSTRUM IS ABSORBED—THIS IS A KEY ISSUE.

Eclectic Medicine: The Holistic Veterinarian

The practice of holistic veterinary medicine is becoming increasingly popular. Practitioners of human and veterinary medicine are integrating natural medicine into conventional medicine. As the scientific basis and benefits of holistic approaches becomes clear, a greater shift towards natural health care will occur in this millennium.

This book has focused on the use of nutraceuticals, which are only one important component of holistic veterinary care. Holistic care defies simple definition. It embraces many eclectic practices including nutritional, herbal, lifestyle, biomechanical and bioenergetic therapies. Specific disciplines such as homeopathy and acupuncture feature strongly in the complementary armamentarium of the holistic vet. Whilst controversies about the safety and effectiveness of treatments exist between the orthodox and the holistic vet, these differences of opinion are rapidly diminishing. The age of holistic care has dawned and pluralistic medicine (medical pluralism) is the thing of the future.

Nature's answers for health lie in the system of balance that we see all around us. Consider, for instance, homeostasis – the state of equilibrium in the body. Homeostasis maintains balance in various functions and in the chemical compositions of fluids and tissues. Physiological and biochemical actions within each organism return that organism to "normal" conditions. To maintain normal body temperature, the body perspires and cools down or generates goose pimples and shivers to warm up. When people are diseased or stressed or very old or very young, balance cannot be achieved as quickly.

Nature has provided a system of balance by which a person or a living thing can heal itself – up to a point. There is a limit beyond which healing cannot occur or is incomplete – that is when the

Paracelsian concept of the "external physician" comes into play. Many scientists today believe that the Earth is also a giant, living organism that experiences balance. Nature's system of balance permits the Earth to heal itself according to what is termed the Gaia principle, named for the Greek goddess who became the mother of the Titans and the Cyclopes – the Earth Mother. Some of the best examples of the Earth Mother's protective system can be found in the plant kingdom, which produce vital nutrients, and herbal or botanical compounds.

The re-establishment of a man-nature team may restore balance and health to Earth and its inhabitants, but restoration of harmony does not require that we abandon the trappings of modern society. We know modern technology will play a vital role in bringing health to the planet. Technology that can reveal how, when, and why biochemical messages are carried to and "turn on" cellular particles will help us find the answers that nature holds.

The treatment efficacy of various herbs and nutrients is already being demonstrated by the modern scientific methodology called signal transduction technology. In studies using this technology, concentrates of several herbs have been shown to have very specific effects on the transfer of cellular messages. This research has centered on certain enzymes that play a vital role in coordinating the process of cell proliferation, which is at the heart of the cause of cancer and immune diseases. The ability to see inside of cells will radically alter the use of natural medicines and result in an "herbal revolution".

Choosing your parents wisely!

In this book, we have focused on the importance of nutrition and remedies of natural origin for maintaining wellness in our beloved companion animals. Whilst this approach is a key step in health maintenance, genetics and hereditary factors play a significant role in the health of a pet throughout his or her life. In order to impress upon people the importance of good breeding for healthy pets, we have mentioned the impossible idea that one can choose one's own parents. As strange as this concept may appear to human beings, it is applicable to companion animals. Therefore, anyone considering owning a pet or having problems with their pet should consider obtaining advice from both breeders and vets. There are many sources of desirable pets and prospective animal owners should go to professional breeders to obtain a pet. Many resources on the internet exist and in the case of dogs, readers are referred to www.hund.ch, where international lists of clubs, services and breeders exist.

As we draw to a close on our discussion of nutraceutical technology, we want every reader to "Love their pet and visit their vet." A reader that is looking for a practitioner of holistic vetinary medicine is referred to search the internet (web) page of www.naturesbenefit.com.

LOVE YOUR PET
AND
VISIT YOUR VET

Resources And Suggested Reading (Books)

Allport RB, *Heal Your Cat the Natural Way*, Reed International Books, NY, 1997.

Allport RB, *Heal Your Dog the Natural Way*, Reed International Books, NY, 1997.

Anderson N, and Peiper H, *Are You Poisoning Your Pets?* Garden City Park, NY, Avery Publishing Group, 1998.

Anderson N, and Peiper H, *Super Nutrition for Animals*, Garden City Park, NY, Avery Publishing Group, 1996.

Belfield, Wendell O, DVM and Zucker M, *The Very Healthy Cat Book: A Vitamin and Mineral Program for Optimal Feline Health*. New York, McGraw-Hill, 1988.

Castelman M, *The Healing Herbs: The Ultimate Guide to the Curative Power of Nature's Medicines*, Emmaus, Pa: Rodale Press, 1991.

Coulter AH, *Alternative Veterinary Medicine Provides Relief for Pets, Alternative and Complementary Therapies*, Vol. 2,4, 245-252, 1996.

DeBairacli Levy J, *Cats Naturally: Natural Rearing for Healthier Domestic Cats*, New York: Faber & Faber, 1991.

DeBairacli Levy J, *The Complete Herbal Handbook for the Dog and Cat*, New York, Faber & Faber, 1991.

Frazier A with Eckroate N, *The New Natural Cat: A Complete Guide for Finicky Owners*, New York: Penguin Books, 1990.

Gfeller RW, DVM and Messonier SR, DVM, *Handbook of Small Animal Toxicology and Poisonings*, Saint Louis, MO, Mosby, 1998.

Goldstein M, DVM, *The Nature of Animal Healing: The Path to Your Pet's Healing, Happiness, and Longevity*, New York: Knopf, New York, 1999.

Humphries J., *Dr. Jim's Animal Clinic for Dogs*, Howell Book House, NY, 1994.

Holt S., *Natural Ways to Digestive Health*, M. Evans and Co. Inc., NY, NY, 2000.

Holt S., *The Natural Way to a Healthy Heart*, M. Evans and Co. Inc., NY, NY, 1999.

Holt S., Barilla J., *The Power of Cartilage*, Kensington US, NY, NY, 1998.

Holt S., *The Soy Revolution*, Dell, Random House Inc., NY, NY, 1999.

Holt S., Comac L. *Miracle Herbs*, Birch Lane Press (www.well-nesspublishing.com) 1997.

Irlbeck NA, *Nutrition and Care of Animals*, Dubuque, Iowa: Kendall/Hunt Publishing, 1996.

Jacob SW, Lawrence RM, Zucker M, *The Miracle of MSM: The Natural Solution for Pain*, G. Putnam's Sons, Penguin Putnam, 1999.

Lazarus P, *Keep Your Pet Healthy the Natural Way*, Indianapolis: Macmillan, 1983.

Messonier S., *The Arthritis Solution for Dogs*. Prima Pets, Prima Publishing, Roseville, Ca, 2000.

Monti DJ, *Human and Animal Medicine Meet on the Bridge*, News Section, Journal of the American Veterinary Medical Association, 217, No 12, pp. 1775 –8, 2000.

Norsworthy GD and Fooshee SK, *Ask the Vet: Questions and Answers for Dog Owners*, Guelph, Ontario, Canada: Lifelarn, 1997.

Patmore A and Couzens T, *Your Natural Dog: A guide to Behavior and Health Care*, New York: Carroll & Graf Publishers, 1998.

Pitcairn Rtl., Pitcairn Stl., *Dr. Pitcairn's Complete Guide to Natural Health for Dogs and Cats*, Rodale Press Inc., Emmaus, PA, 1995.

Puotinen CJ, *The Encyclopedia of Natural Pet Care*, Keats Publishing, New Canaan, CT. (McGraw Hill), 1998.

Reavley N., *New Encyclopedia Vitamins, Minerals, Supplements and Herbs*, M. Evans and Co. Inc., NY, NY 1998.

Schoen AM, DVM, *Love, Miracles, and Animal Healing*, New York: Simon & Schuster, 1997.

Schoen AM, Wynn SG. (editors), *Complementary and Alternative Veterinary Medicine: Principles and Practice*, Mosby Inc., St. Louis, Times Mirror Company, 1998.

Self, HP, *A Modern Horse Herbal*. Addington, Buckingham, England: Kenilworth Press, 1996.

Siegal M and Cornell University. *The Cornell Book of Cats*, New York: Villard Books, 1989.

Siegal M and the School of Veterinary Medicine, University of California at Davis, *UC Davis Books of Dogs*, New York: HarperCollins Publishers, 1995.

Stein D, *The Natural Remedy Book for Dogs and Cats*, Freedom, Calif: Crossing Press, 1994.

Stein D., *The Natural Remedy Book for Dogs and Cats*, The Crossing Press, Freedom CA, 1994.

Tyler VE, Ph.D. Herbs of Choice: *The Therapeutic Use of Phytomedicinals*, Binghamton, NY: Pharmaceutical Products Press, 1994.

Volhard, W and Brown K, DVM, *The Holistic Guide for a Healthy Dog*, New York: Howell Book House, 1995.

Wolff HG, DVM, *Your Healthy Cat: Homeopathic Medicines for Common Feline Ailments.* Berkely, Calif.: North Atlantic Books, 1991.

Wulff-Tilford M and Tilford GL, *Herbal Remedies for Dogs and Cats: A Pocket Guide to Selection and Use.* Connor, Mont: Mountain Weed Publishing, 1997.

Wulff- Tilford ML, Tilford GL, *All You Ever Wanted to Know About Herbs for Pets*, Bowtie Press Inc., Irvine California, 1999.

www.wellnesspublishing.com

Yamall, C, *Cat Care Naturally.* New York: Charles E. Tuttle, 1995.

WEB SITES

www.naturesbenefit.com (commercial)
www.enaturalhealth.com (education)
www.altvetmed.com (education, holistic care)
www.naturalpetshealth.com (education)
www.naturalvethealth.com (education)
www.naturalantiangiogenesis.com (education)
www.wellnesspublishing.com (books)
www.nzymes.com (commercial)
www.daneworld.com (commercial)

USEFUL SOURCES OF INFORMATION OBTAINED BY EMAIL QUESTIONS

info@naturesbenefit.com (general product info)
GrDaneLady@aol.com (breeder and nutrition advice)
danelady@gsinet.net (breeder and nutrition advice)
stan@nzymes.com (general product info)
jeanette@naturespharmacy.com (product info and nutrition advice)
admin@hund.ch (international contacts, breeders etc.)
drb@deanbaderdvm.com (expert veterinarian advice)
pawsreflect@earthlink.com (product info and nutrition advice)

About the Authors

Stephen Holt, MD, FACP, FACN, FRCP(C), FACG, MRCP (UK) is a medical practitioner in New York. He is a best-selling author and he holds senior academic appointments. Dr. Holt is a frequent guest lecturer at international scientific meetings and he is a popular media expert on health.

Other books by Dr. Holt

The Soy Revolution, Dell Publishing, Random House, NY, NY, 2000.
Natural Ways to Digestive Health, M. Evans Inc., NY, NY, 2000.
The Soy Lifestyle, Wellness Publishing.com, NJ, 2000.
The Natural Way to a Healthy Heart, M. Evans Inc., NY, NY, 1999.
Miracle Herbs with Linda Comac, Carol Publishing, Secaucus, NJ, 1998.
The Power of Cartilage, Kensington, Zebra Books, NY, NY, 1998.
Soya for Health, M. A. Liebert Publishing, Larchmont, NY, 1997.
The Alcohol Clinical Index with H. A. Skinner, Addiction Research Foundation Press, Toronto, Canada, 1983.

Dean R. Bader, DVM is a practitioner of holistic and conventional veterinary medicine. He has many years of experience in animal care and practices at Shingle Springs Veterinary Clinic in Shingle Springs, CA.

Special note to readers: PLEASE READ

This book focuses on specific nutraceutical technologies for health maintenance. The word "nutraceutical" (or nutriceutical) is used to describe the use of nutrients as agents to promote health and wellness. Descriptions of nutraceuticals have been extended from nutrients to herbs, plant extracts and plant chemicals. The authors present a new perspective to bring human nutraceutical advances to veterinary medicine. The authors are not giving treatment advice, they are discussing the development of a range of nutraceutical formulations with potential application in the veterinary field. Practitioners of human medicine are not licensed to treat animals (pets), in the same way that veterinarians are not licensed to treat humans.

The American Veterinary Medical Association (AVMA) has issued guidelines for the practice of alternative and complementary (or pluralistic) medicine for animals. Any treatment of pets should at least be performed under the supervision of or by referral from a licensed veterinarian who is providing concurrent care. The authors are not making treatment claims, they are discussing an interpretation of medical and veterinary literature. More extensive discussions of holistic veterinary care should be accessed before pet owners decide on non-conventional treatments for their animals (see resources section 12).

The American Veterinary Medical Association (AVMA) has summarized the science of nutraceutical medicine in the following definition: *"Nutraceutical medicine is the use of micronutrients, macronutrients, and other supplements as therapeutic agents"*. The AVMA stresses that: *"Communication on the potential risks and benefits from the use of these compounds within the context of a valid veterinarian/client/patient relationship is important. Continued research and education on the use of nutraceuticals in veterinary medicine is advised. Care must be taken with the use of herbs and botanicals in pets"*.

The authors support the viewpoint of the AVMA and recommends that the guidance of a licensed veterinarian is required before pets are "treated". However, optimal nutrition and beneficial alteration of body functions fall within the category of dietary supplements in humans and food supplements in pets. Dietary supplements cannot be used to diagnose, treat or prevent any disease. The authors stress that they are not offering treatment advice with nutraceuticals for pets.

The following disclaimer is applied to this book. The ideas and advice in this book are based upon the experiences and training of the authors. The authors have provided their own interpretation of literature and opinions are divided on the value of nutraceuticals that are used for the maintenance of well-being. The suggestions in this book are definitely not meant to be a substitute for a careful evaluation and treatment of a pet by a *licensed veterinarian*.

Many nutraceuticals may interact with existing therapies administered by a veterinarian and disclosure of nutraceutical use in the vet/client/patient relationship is mandatory. The authors do not recommended changing or adding medication or dietary supplements (nutraceuticals) in the presence of significant disease, without consulting a veterinarian. The authors specifically disclaim any liability arising directly or indirectly from the use of this book, which focuses on a specific series of remedies of natural origin.

None of the statements made in this book have been approved by any regulatory agency or academic institution. The remedies described or their components are not drugs and they have not been approved for diagnosis, prevention or treatment of any disease. Not all herbs, botanicals or nutrients are approved feed ingredients.

The contents of this book focus on dogs, cats and horses, recognizing that these animals have special, species-specific and "individualized" needs. The suggestions in this book must not be applied to exotic pets. <u>Again, it must be stressed that only a veterinarian has the training to address the specific, health needs of animals.</u> Needs of pets vary greatly by species.